Contents

Contributors

Viv Allison, SRN, RSCN, Paediatric Oncology Outreach Nurse Specialist (POONS), Newcastle, UK

Lucy Andrews, RGN, RN Child, BSc (Hons), Community Children's Nurse, Cambridgeshire, UK

Joanna Assey, MSc, BN (Hons) Child Branch, BSc (Hons), RMN, RN Child Branch, ENMH, Senior Clinical Nurse Specialist working with children who have a learning disability, Dorset Healthcare Foundation Trust, Bournemouth, UK

Trish Bannister, Regional Cleft Lip and Palate Service, North West of England, UK

Amber Barnum, RN Child, Community Children's Staff Nurse, Cambridgeshire, UK

Jo Bennett, RGN, RSCN, MSc Advanced Practice, PGDip/Cert Advanced Practice, BSc (Hons), DPSN, CMS, APLS, Advanced Paediatric Nurse Practitioner, Children's Services, Walsall Hospitals NHS Trust, Walsall, UK

Peter Callery, BA (Hons), RGN, RSCN, MSc, PhD, Chair in Children's Nursing, School of Nursing, Midwifery and Social Work, University of Manchester, Manchester, UK

Anne Casey, RSCN, MSc, FRCN, Editor, Paediatric Nursing, Journal Royal College of Nursing, RCN Publishing Company, Harrow, Middlesex, UK

Hazel Chamberlain, RGN, RSCN, BSc (Hons) Nursing, MA Child Protection, Lead Nurse Specialist in Child Protection, Central Manchester and Manchester Children's University Hospitals NHS Trust, Manchester, UK

Janice Christie, PhD, MA, BSc, PGCHET, RN, RSCPHN, Teaching Fellow, School of Nursing and Midwifery, Queen's University, Belfast, Northern Ireland, UK

Pat Coldicutt, BA (Hons), DPSN, RGN, RSCN, ENB 216, ENB 998, ENB N100, C&G 7307, CNS Stoma Care/Promotion of Continence, Royal Liverpool Children's NHS Trust, Liverpool, UK

Christine English, RGN, RSCN, DPSN, BSc (Hons), MSc, PGDE, Matron/Senior Lecturer – joint post, Newcastle upon Tyne Hospitals NHS Foundation Trust and Northumbria University, UK

Jane Farrell, RGN/RSCN, A50 Diploma – Paediatric Community Nursing, NARTC – Paediatric Respiratory ENB N83, Children's Asthma Nurse Specialist, Heywood, Middleton and Rochdale Primary Care Trust, Lancashire, UK

Carole Gelder, RGN, RSCN, BA (Hons), PG Diploma in Health Professional Education (Lecturer), MSc Health Professional Education, Lecturer/Practitioner/Children's Diabetes Nurse Specialist, Leeds University/St James University Hospital and Leeds General Infirmary, UK

Gill Gibson, Formerly Clinical Nurse Specialist – Children's Learning Disability, The Tree House, Stockport Foundation Trust

Alan Glasper, BA (Hons), PhD, RSCN, RGN, ONC, DN (Lond), Cert Ed RNT, Professor of Children's and Young People's Nursing, University of Southampton, Southampton, UK

Viv Hall, RCN, RM, BSc, MSc, ANNP, Lead ANNP for the Greater Manchester Neonatal Transport Service (GMNeTS), St Mary's Hospital for Women and Children, Manchester, UK

Cathy Harrington, BSc (Child Health), Paediatric Cardiac Liaison Sister, Bristol Children's Hospital, Bristol, UK

Jane Hughes, School of Nursing, Midwifery and Health Visiting, University of Manchester, Manchester, UK

Liz Hutchinson, MSc, RGN, RSCN, DN Cert, Nottingham Children and Young People's Rheumatology Service, Nottingham, UK

Jeremy Jolley, BN, MA, PhD, PGCEA, PGC Theol, SRN, RSCN, Senior Lecturer, The University of Hull, Hull, UK

Bernadette Lee, RGN/RSCN, Oncology 237, Diploma in Aromatherapy Massage, Diploma in Epilepsy, Paediatric Epilepsy Nurse Specialist, Stepping Hill Hospital, Stockport, UK

Geraldine Lyte, School of Nursing, Midwifery and Health Visiting, University of Manchester, Manchester, UK

Amy Martin-Long, Diploma in Health/Registered Nurse (Child), BSc (Hons), Specialist Practitioner in Child Health, MSC Autonomous Practice in Minor Injury and Illness (60 credits outstanding), Paediatric Sister, Manchester Royal Infirmary Children's Accident and Emergency, Central Manchester and Manchester Children's University Hospitals NHS Trust, Manchester, UK

Sarah Moxon, BNurs (Hons) Child, Staff Nurse (Band 5), Neonatal Intensive Care, Great Ormond Street Hospital for Children, London, UK

Barry Nixon, RGN, RNMH, LD, RMN, DipN, National Workforce Lead, CAMHS, Higher Ince, Wigan, UK

Jackie Parkes, PhD, BNurs (Hons), RGN, RSCN, NDN Cert, PGCHET, Senior Lecturer in Children's Nursing, School of Nursing and Midwifery, Queen's University, Belfast, Northern Ireland, UK

Jayne Price, RGN, RN (Child), BSc (Hons), MSC, PG Dip Ed (Nursing), Senior Teaching Fellow (Children's Nursing), Queen's University, Belfast, Northern Ireland, UK

Jim Richardson, BA, RGN, RSCN, PGCE, PhD, Head of Division (Family Care), Faculty of Health, Sport and Science, University of Glamorgan, Wales, UK

Susie Tinsley, RN(LD), Dip SW, Specialist Nurse (Learning Disability), Children's LD Team, Tree House Children's Centre, Stockport Foundation Trust

Alison Twycross, PhD, MSc, DMS, CertEd (HE), RGN, RMN, RSCN, Principal Lecturer in Children's Nursing, Kingston University and St George's University of London, London, UK

Foreword

Putting our own lives in the hands of a health professional is unnerving – so how much more terrifying is handing over the lives or welfare of our children? Every working day children's nurses accept the honour of being that trusted professional, the obligation of doing the right thing for that child, young person, family and indeed society. However brief the encounter, however limited the contact, whatever particular challenges face a child or family, every word, every action, must maximise every child's life and living potential and must, for society, enhance the health and well-being of children and young people in whose hands lie the future. Whatever nursing position held or whatever role performed, all nurses involved have accepted the responsibility to keep their own knowledge, skills and competence up-to-date and to develop nursing practice for the benefit of their young clients.

This book offers a unique insight into current, professional practice for children's nurses. It has been written specifically for all nurses, student nurses and support staff, who care for children and young people and who want to consider the scope of their current or future practice potential. Looking towards the future does not, however, negate the need to learn from our past and children's nurses have built with pride on the traditions of dedicated predecessors. These forerunners, viewed as nurses of 'sick' children, were only too aware of the impact of environmental and societal factors upon children's health. They saw clearly that public health and the promotion of good child rearing practices were core elements of their practice.

In 2008 sickness, high technology interventions and hospital-based acute care are no longer viewed as the sole focus of children's nurses. Children's nursing roles are increasingly appearing in primary care settings and discussions will continue around ensuring that professionals are appropriately educated and prepared to meet the needs of children and young people. This of course extends beyond the delivery of care in hospitals to include new ambulatory centres, polyclinics and indeed at any point of access for a child. It may be reassuring to insist that all nursing staff who work with children and young people in any setting are children's nurses. This, however, is unrealistic, restricting the flexibility of the health workforce; for example, some employers are enthusiastic about the employment of generic nursing staff in primary care and access areas, who can then care for adults and children. This is a challenge for children's nurses, who will all too eagerly share subjective outcomes that they believe support the qualitative value of their role. What is actually required, however, is measures of effectiveness such as prevention of admission or reduced length of stay or reduced drug expenditure. Best practice in children's nursing practice is no longer limited to clinical effectiveness and meeting patient expectations but cost effectiveness and intelligent use of available resources that more children can benefit from our limited health service budget.

Best use of resources and good outcomes for children, young people and families are indeed what are aimed for in any organisation. This leads to consideration as to who is available to provide care: clarity around care required is certainly the starting point and then these needs can be matched to the competence of available staff or competences that will need to be developed. What is important for the safety of the children and young people is a realistic basis for competence development which takes into account not only the required knowledge and skills but also the professional accountability of staff being accepted or developed to provide that particular aspect of care. For example, if assistant roles are developed, competences required should be agreed, developed and assessed but with clarity around what is not accepted due to a lack of underpinning knowledge or formal professional accountability. This is as true for nursing assistants as for nurses developing advanced practice that will never be, and should not seek to be, mini doctors but, within the confines of their professional accountability, will be maxi nurses.

Evidence of effectiveness of nursing developments, in terms of the impact upon patient outcomes and service delivery, will be increasingly important and children's nurses need to capitalise on funded opportunities to undertake research that will provide a defensible evidence base for development in nursing practice with children and young people. The development of children's nurses requires good practice from children's nursing leaders and in 2008 this necessarily includes a level of business and political acumen that will support others in making a case for change that meets the demands of today's health service. What is required from clinicians, managers, educationalists and policy makers is a shared passion for children's nursing with a total commitment to maximising the potential of this dedicated and proud workforce. This book sets out the bases of children's nursing for nurses, students and support staff who not only care for children, young people and their families in today's healthcare settings, but who will also help to determine the future of our young profession.

Professor Judith Ellis MBE
Director of Nursing, Education and Workforce Development
Great Ormond Street Hospital, London

Preface

Child health care has been evolving over the last 20 years to such an extent that the scope and practice of children's nursing cannot be considered in the same way as it was historically. Among the many challenges facing modern day children's nurses are changes that have arisen since the publication of the Children's National Service Framework (DH 2004). The emergence of assistant and advanced practitioner roles is another major consideration, as well as factors such as recognition of the transitional needs of young people as they emerge into adulthood. This book aims to present the scope of both current and developing practice of nurses who care for children and young people (CYP).

This book includes interdisciplinary approaches to CYP health care. Not only does it acknowledge joint working in the interests of children and families, but also the diversity of the approaches used to include children, young people, parents and significant others in the care process. It also includes the most recent guiding policies and reflects demographic changes and strategic developments in the current National Health Service (NHS). Case studies and commentaries from leading practitioners, educators and policy makers have been included in many of the chapters, for example the experiences of newly qualified nurses in Chapters 4 and 5.

Jane Hughes
Geraldine Lyte

Part 1
Becoming a Children's Nurse: An Exploration of Developing Scope and Practice

Introduction

Geraldine Lyte

Part 1 of this book focuses on the emergence and evolvement of children's nursing role in health care. Child health care has been evolving over the past 20 years to such an extent that the scope and practice of children's nursing cannot be considered in the same way as it was done historically. Among the many challenges facing modern day children's nurses are changes that have arisen since the publication of the Children's National Service Framework (DH 2004) and Every Child Matters (DH 2004). The emergence of assistant and advanced practitioner roles is another major consideration, as well as factors such as recognition of the transitional needs of young people as they emerge into adulthood. This book aims to present the scope of both current and developing practice of nurses who care for children and young people.

In Chapter 1, Jeremy Jolley presents an overview of historical and contemporary events and developments that have shaped the role of children's and young people's nurses, and associated support roles, for the 21st century. This sets the scene for further historical analyses of children's nursing role in later chapters, such as that provided by Barry Nixon in Chapter 7, as part of his review of children's and adolescents' mental health services. In Chapter 2, Alan Glasper and Jim Richardson focus on professional education issues, early professional practice and particular knowledge and skills needed by children's nurses. They include an analysis of the future direction for children's nursing education which has recently been debated within the profession. Part 1 concludes with Chapter 3, in which Anne Casey offers a comparison of children's nursing roles in a variety of international settings.

Chapter 1
The Emergence of the 21st Century Children's Nurse

Jeremy Jolley

Introduction

You will be reading this book because you are interested in current issues in children's nursing. Perhaps you wish to keep up to date with issues in nursing practice or perhaps you are learning how to be a children's nurse. In any case, your key orientation is likely to be your practice in a range of health care settings with children and young people (CYP), their families and others who are important to them. Why start this book with an account of the history of children's nursing? Answering this question is based on an appreciation that children's nursing is more than a job, it is a profession. As professional people, nurses have a sense of responsibility for their discipline because in a real sense it belongs to them. This includes how the discipline is developing, progressing and moving forward. Nurses increasingly direct their practice, for example, through analysis and application of the best available evidence and by developing and changing practice to maximise the quality of care which they and others deliver.

What is children's nursing?

Following on from this, children's nursing is a professional activity which is focused on the delivery of care to CYP with a range of health care needs. It embraces the inclusion and involvement of families and significant others in that care, according to the needs and wishes of the CYP concerned. Childhood spans the most important period in our lives, incorporating birth and those babies born prematurely, infancy, being a toddler and then a young child, older children, early adolescence and the transition of young people into adulthood.

Children's nurses provide health care to CYP at home, at school, in primary care settings and in hospitals. Their practice is based on wide ranging skills and knowledge such as managing psychological as well as physical trauma, spirituality and care of the dying, and the science of maintaining body systems to sustain life. Children's nurses also work with adults in family units and other carer settings and of course in collaboration with other disciplines. The role of a children's nurse, as it lies in juxtaposition between parent/carer and child, is one that is ancient in its history, professional in its continuous search for better care, and privileged beyond measure.

Why history?

Children's nursing today encompasses a modern, caring discipline which embraces technical and scientific knowledge. It is also a discipline which has a long and interesting history, practiced over the centuries by women and men, by the rich and the poor and by the educated and uneducated (Evans 2004, Wyman 1984). It is important to have some appreciation of this colourful history because children's nurses can learn much that is useful today from the knowledge of good and poor practices recorded in history. In order to improve or develop children's nursing, for example, understanding from where it has come is as important as what is happening currently. It places today's practice into perspective and can even help to determine ways in which current practice can be improved. It can help you develop a plan for how you wish to develop children's nursing in your own lifetime. Perhaps, at no other time in modern history have we needed knowledge of the history of nursing as much as we do today. This chapter will aim to put the rest of the book into perspective for you.

Child health care before 1852

The nursing care of children has taken place in every age and in every society (Cunningham 1995). For as long as there have been children there have been those who have been ill and who have been injured. It would be incorrect to assume that the care of children is necessarily better today than it was in the past. Instead, you might question notions of an increasing degree of human civilisation, of children having a harder time than today, and of historical cruelty (Jolley 2006b). Some authors have argued that the care of children has consistently improved as civilisation has developed (e.g. Aries 1962, DeMause 1974); however, it is important to consider the evidence carefully before accepting this argument (Jolley 2006b). On the other hand, the presence of war and famine in our own time offer testament to the way in which children are not always seen as a priority. Overall though, there is overwhelming evidence from history that parents and others tried hard to keep their children in good health (Hardyment 1995).

Little is known of nursing that must have taken place before Britain's medieval period. Nurses and those who cared for sick children rarely kept records of the activities and most of the documentation if any were lost. Some records remain from the great centres of civilisation in Greece (*ca.* 400 years BC), the Egyptian civilisation from the time of the Pharaohs and from the ancient

Arabian and Chinese literature (till 1931). It may be surmised however, that much of the great wisdom of the past is lost to us. We do know that the ancient Greek and Arabic texts (written by people such as Hippocrates and Rhazes) were still being used in the 16th century (till 1931, Ellis 2001). Some of the contemporary medical texts in this period still remain today, thanks to the fact that printing had become available. Nevertheless it should not be assumed that these early authors were 'doctors' and that they therefore belong to the history of medicine. Thomas Phaer's text of 1545 is as much about nursing as it is about medicine (Bowers 1999, Jolley 2006a). Perhaps, it is only from the 18th and 19th centuries that medicine and nursing begin to be considered separate disciplines as we know them today.

Monastic and religious nursing orders

Many of us are familiar with the ruined monasteries and abbeys in the British towns and countryside. From the 4th and 5th centuries until the dissolution of the monasteries by Henry VIII, some of these large institutions provided a degree of nursing for the traveller and for those in the local community (Evans 2004). Baly (1995) pointed out that some of the religious orders such as those of St. Benedict and St. Augustine tended to provide a service to the community, while others such as the Carthusians and Cistercians were more enclosed. A number of these orders provided a service to specific groups of people, for example, the St. Antonines provided care to the mentally ill (Mackintosh 1997). However, there is little evidence of the provision of children's nursing by the monasteries and it is therefore likely that most of the care they provided was to adult travellers and to pilgrims.

There were also military orders which came about at the time of the Crusades. One of these orders, the Knights of St. John of Jerusalem provided hospital care. The ruins of their hospitals can still be found today in Malta and in Rhodes (Baly 1995). Again, however, most of their patients would have been travellers and there is very little indication that they provided care to sick children. The Knights of St. John of Jerusalem live on in the UK today as the St. John's Ambulance Brigade and members wear the badge of the order (a Maltese Cross) on their uniform.

So it can be surmised that the monastic movement did not make a sizable contribution to the history of children's nursing. There existed no institutionalised discipline that focused its work on the needs of sick children. Of course, one should not conclude from this that children did not receive nursing and medical treatment. Instead, that medical and nursing knowledge which existed at the time is likely to have been common knowledge and delivered by the child's family. What advice that was available would probably have been acquired from local people, those with experience of the particular disorder and, where such contacts existed, from those who were better educated. In this way, nursing knowledge was much more a part of the *common understanding* than is the case today.

Families consequently provided the main care and treatment for sick children. They would have *known* how to do this and would not necessarily have been dependent on people with greater knowledge. Today, families still provide much of the health care required by their CYP but they have a range of expert care providers available such as those found in today's hospitals. This notion of *expert* is quite modern. Experts can, of course, be very useful but their introduction into society has removed a significant part of the traditional role of the family particularly in health care and education.

It is also interesting that it was largely men who worked as nurses in the monastic and military models of health care that were prevalent until the dissolution of the monasteries in the reign of Henry VIII.

With the passing of the monastic movement, health care was largely un-institutionalised and became the responsibility of the individual family. On the whole, general hospitals did not begin to develop until the 18th century (Evans 2004) and these did relatively little work with children. However, the general hospitals of the 18th and 19th centuries were working to a very different model and were institutional in the separation of Medicine and Nursing. In the days of the monasteries, the distinction between care and treatment had been relatively indistinct. In the mid-19th century, however, Florence Nightingale built on separate models of nursing and medicine at a time when roles of men and women were particularly distinct. So, Nursing became an almost exclusively female activity and Medicine almost exclusively male. This model was so integrated with societal notions of the proper roles of men and women that it did not begin to be overturned until the middle of the 20th century, and then only very slowly.

Today, it is accepted that women have much to offer in Medicine and men have much to offer in Nursing. It cannot now be doubted that health care would be impoverished without the respective contribution of men and women in today's health care professions.

The Renaissance

Medicine and nursing have not always been scientific disciplines. In common with his peers, Thomas Phaer (1510–1560) believed that God had endowed nature with healing powers (Jolley 2006a). This did not just apply to drugs obtained from plants and so on but also to a range of other materials. Phaer recommends the use of an amulet (a charm) for the treatment of childhood epilepsy:

> I fynde that manye thynges have a naturall vertue agaynste the fallyng evell, not of any quality elemental but by a simgular propertie, or rather an influence of heaven, whyche almyghtye God hath gyven into thynges here in earth … These (red coral, sapphires or stones from a swallows stomach), or one of them, hanged about the necke o the childe saveth and preserveth it from the sayde syckenes (p. 41).

It is not surprising that many of the children Phaer cared for had diseases we would recognise today. Here he informs his reader of how to recognise the dangerous condition of epiglottis:

> [It is a] daungerous syckenes bothe in yonge and olde, called in Latyne angina. It is an inflammation of the necke with swellying and great peyne. Somtyme it lyeth in the verye throte upon the wesent pipe, and then it is excedying perillous for it stoppeth the breath and straguleth the pacient anone … The signes are apparaunt to syght, and besydes that the chylde can not crye, nether swallowe downe hys meat and drynke wythout payne (p. 54).

Phaer also writes about the care of the child with the lethal condition of Small Pox; his treatment seems particularly holistic and caring. Firstly, he declares that there is no effective treatment and cautions against the use of treatment that may make the child worse:

> The best and most sure helpe in this case is not to meddle wyth any kynde of medicines, but to let nature woorke her operation (p. 61).

Phaer suggests some medicine to soothe pain: rose or fennel water to soothe the eyes and rose water for the child to gargle with where he or she has oral pain. He was obviously as much concerned with the child's discomfort as he was with providing treatment for the disease. In this regard, indeed Phaer was Britain's first children's nurse.

The majority of this early literature is not specifically focussed on the care of children. Since Phaer did much of his work with sick children, he was almost certainly exceptional in this respect. In fact the first organisation of paediatricians (in the UK) did not become established until 1928 (Forfar *et al.* 1989) and of paediatric surgeons until 1954 (Dunn 2006). Some forms of nursing were controlled by law as early as the 16th century (Bowers 1999) but for the most part there existed no separate organisation of children's nurses until the children's hospitals began to be built from 1852. A register specifically for children's nurses was opened in 1919 and the first national organisation of children's nurses, the Association of British Paediatric Nurses, was established between 1936 and 1938 (Duncombe 1979).

The 17th and 18th centuries

Even during the 17th and 18th centuries there were no hospitals for sick children in Britain, nor was there a formal discipline of children's nursing. However, there were two non-hospital-based models of child care in operation before the mid-19th century; they are the foundling hospitals and the children's dispensaries, which have been seen as precursors to modern children's nursing.

The foundling hospitals

A 'foundling' is an abandoned child (a small thing found). It is sadly the case that in the 18th century many people could not afford to keep their babies and this was especially the case in the rapidly growing cities. Young mothers were often caught in a web of poverty, poor housing and lack of family support. Industrialisation had spawned large, unhealthy towns in which the poor often vainly sought escape from the traditional ways of countryside living. This resulted in the breakdown of the extended family and the support that this had once provided. For the first time in history, people found themselves without the support of their family and local community.

Thomas Coram (1668–1751) was a businessman and shipbuilder who from lowly beginnings had developed trade with New England. Coram was saddened to see the number of dead and dying babies abandoned in the streets of London. He worked for many years to get an official approval and sufficient funding for his 'Darling Project', the opening of the first 'hospital' for foundlings in Britain. His business in New England was eventually to falter, largely because of Coram's relatively poor social position and of the lawless nature of the new American states. In his old age, he saw the opening of the London Foundling Hospital as his most proud achievement. Indeed Wagner (2004, p. 1) suggests that:

> Coram is rightly acclaimed for having forced society, rather against its will, to interest itself in the fate of its youngest, most defenceless, destitute and abandoned citizens.

Coram was, according to Wagner (2004, p. 4), a man *of startling integrity in a corrupted age*. It was indeed this awakening of society to its responsibility towards defenceless children that was to see the development of first the children's dispensaries and later the children's hospitals with which we are familiar today. Arton (1992) suggests that the foundling hospitals, the first of which was opened by Thomas Coram in 1741, were the first real children's hospitals in Britain. It is probably better to consider these as orphanages rather than children's hospitals but they did employ people to care for the children and it is known that many of these children were sick. The main reason for not including the foundling hospitals as part of the history of children's nursing is that the (nursing) staff were never professionally organised. In this way there was never to be a 'discipline' of foundling hospital staff.

The aim of the foundling hospitals was to recover abandoned children and to provide them with accommodation, food and a Christian education. Moreover, the development of the foundling hospitals was noteworthy for two reasons. The first is that some foundling hospitals did in time become children's hospitals. This is the case with what is now Alder Hey Hospital, Liverpool and with L'Hôpital des Enfants Malades (the hospital for sick children) in Paris. It was the existence of L'Hôpital des Enfants Malades that made envious physicians in this country to establish children's hospitals here, in particular Charles West to establish Great Ormond Street Hospital (GOS) in London. However, perhaps the most important reason to consider the foundling hospitals seriously is that they highlight the moment when society accepted responsibility for children in need of care. It was this very awakening that enabled the notion of a hospital for children to be embraced by British society during the 18th century.

The children's dispensaries

George Armstrong (1781) opened the first children's dispensary in 1769 in Red Lion Square, London (Jolley 2007a). The dispensary was rather like hospital outpatient department. Here, working parents (the 'deserving poor') could bring their sick children to obtain advice and medicine from apothecaries (pharmacists) and physicians (though usually the former). Armstrong himself had undergone medical training but was not licensed as a medical practitioner because of his social background (Jolley 2007a). This did not stop him writing two important texts on the treatment of sick children (Armstrong 1771, 1777) in which he took the opportunity to promote his own dispensary.

Armstrong was influential in propagating the then novel idea that children's diseases could be treated successfully. The prevailing belief was that children were too difficult to treat and that (rightly) most treatments of the day were too powerful for children. In one of his texts on paediatric medicine, Armstrong (1777, p. vii) refers to:

> the absurd notion, which has too long, and too universally prevailed, that there is little or nothing to be done in the complaints of children has prevented many parents from applying to physicians for advice.

Armstrong's accounts of the diseases of children are likely to have prompted the medical fraternity that there might be good purpose in developing a new discipline of medicine for children.

Armstrong's dispensary and those that followed provide an important building block in the history of children's nursing. This was a charity-based model of health care which pre-dated the children's hospitals, which provided treatment to sick children. Armstrong spoke out against hospitals as being inappropriate for young children because of the risk of cross-infection and because of the needs of children for their parents. In practice, however, Armstrong was simply trying to promote his own dispensary. This was an endeavour that would eventually fail. Queues of ragged children waiting to see an apothecary simply failed to inspire the wealthy middle- and upper-class benefactors whose financial support was so necessary (Jolley 2007a). The children's dispensaries declined about the time that Charles West was founding the first children's hospital in 1852.

Charles West had worked in a dispensary (the Universal Dispensary in Waterloo Bridge Road, London). However he had learned an important lesson from his work in the dispensaries: health care for children was expensive and therefore required proper funding. To achieve this it was necessary to have the support of the most influential members of society. These people would not only give money, they would give credibility to the scheme and then more money would follow. The hospital provided a romantic image of children's health care that the dispensaries had always lacked. The provision of civilised, educated and humane nursing was an essential element to this romantic image.

The co-dependency of medicine and nursing was now also understood, so paediatric medicine would from now on take an active interest in the development of paediatric nursing. The dispensaries would fail but would spawn the hugely successful children's hospitals. The first children's hospital was opened in Great Ormond Street, London, in 1852. By the end of the same century a children's hospital had been built in almost every large town in Britain; many of these hospitals remain today.

Florence Nightingale's modernisation of nursing was hugely influential in the hospital movement and was based on the traditional Victorian division of labour between men and women and a further division of labour which separated classes of female kind (Mackintosh 1997). It was also dependent on the Victorian notion of 'family' with the male as head and female as carer (Evans 2004). As in the middle-class Victorian household, caring was seen as a simple activity but one which required obedience to the doctor's orders. Nurses needed to be reliable, kind, honest and with enough wit to follow orders. For this reason and from this point forward women were to dominate nursing, military obedience was replaced by the discipline of the household servant and planning and problem solving was left to (male) physicians and surgeons. At least this model allowed for the nursing of sick children. Based on such a model children's hospitals were founded and children's nursing as a discipline was born.

From 1852 to 1918: The romantic years

What makes the beginning of hospital nursing different from the informal care of sick children that had taken place before is that children's nurses began to see themselves as an occupational and later a professional entity. They began to work as an occupational unit and with an overall sense of responsibility, not only for the children for whom they were caring but for the discipline of children's nursing as a whole. This is still very much the case today, with children's nurses as members of a profession and carrying responsibilities not only to the CYP entrusted to their care but also to the wider profession. In this way, children's nurses have cultivated a responsibility to study, to improve their collective understanding and application of nursing, to conduct and/or implement research and to publish ideas about how they can continue to improve what they do.

This sense of responsibility to CYP and their families is evident from the beginning. Charles West established a set of 'rules' for the GOS. These rules were copied by every other children's hospital because GOS was used as a template for hospitals that developed after it. West's rules for nurses can easily be misunderstood today. Nurses were to be kind, respectful and honourable. They were to show respect for physicians and always recognise that the physician had a better knowledge of medicine than did the nurse (West 1854). However, all professional groups have rules that define their professional status. What matters here is that nurses accepted these rules for themselves; they accepted 'standards' both of practice and of their relationship with physicians. This relationship was mutually respectful and employed the middle-class values of the day. Physicians such as Charles West now understood that they needed nurses and so began an unusually cooperative relationship between two professional groups and one that is still very much in existence today.

In two letters to the Times, Sir James Paget, one of the founding fathers of modern medicine, writes of nurses, that they were:

> kind, loving, holistic, but simple people whom men would do well to emulate'. And that 'There were no such nurses … especially for children, as women' Men (doctors), however clever, were apt to be too studious, to treat their patients as different cases, the singularity of which occupied all their attention. But it was not so with women (nurses). Their skill was subordinate to their love, and men would do well to emulate them in their gentleness, their tenderness, and their watchfulness (Paget 1874).

Of course nursing was a very new discipline at this time, its members were recruited largely from the servant classes. Nevertheless, and much to the credit of these early nurses, they won the respect of some of the most well regarded physicians and surgeons in the country (Jolley 2007b).

The needs of children for their parents and for play and respect for children as children were well understood and soon became integrated in the nurses' practice (Jolley 2006c). Cruelty, even overt unkindness, to CYP was not tolerated in this period. Records from Yorkhill hospital show that nurses were dismissed if they hit a child (Yorkhill Hospitals Archive 1916–1932) and were also dismissed if they showed an inability to keep children happy and to communicate effectively with them as children. At the end of the 19th century Catherine Wood (Wood 1888, Jolley 2006c), Lady Superintendent of GOS, gave an account of children's nursing that seems perfectly relevant today:

> Order and discipline there must be, or the children will not be happy; but the Ward that is tidied up to perfection, in which the little ones look like well drilled soldiers, when the home look of liberty is absent, and nothing is out of its place, is hardly suggestive of the happy heart of a child. Toys and games are as much part of the treatment as physic, and the ceaseless chatter and careless distribution of the toys are surely consistent with a well-ordered children's Ward. As a convalescent, a child requires nearly as much attention as one in bed, and because the heart of a child is set on mischief, certainly as much looking after. Some of the older children may make themselves of use in the Ward; but also they may be a great deal of trouble, so that from first to last the sick child is some person's care (p. 508).

> Over and above the actual skilled Nursing, it is necessary to develop in the Nurse the mother's instinct, the grand self-sacrifice and self-forgetfulness that are the outcome of the mother's love; we want each Nurse to gather her little

ones into her arms with the resolve that she will spend and be spent for them. They are hers, and for a time they will look to her for a mother's love and a mother's care. They must be more than cases to her, or they will not thrive as they might in her care. Let us put into the arms of a young Nurse some poor little neglected babe. It is to be her charge by day, and she is to do her best with it; her pride will be aroused, especially if some other young Nurse also has a case, and a generous rivalry between the two will be to the manifest advantage of the babes. Suppose that this babe improves in the marvellous way that babes do, with love and intelligent care, then that Nurse will have learnt a lesson in the care of young infants that will abide by her always (p. 509).

This first period in children's nursing's history was a romantic one. There are many reasons for this but here it is sufficient to note that the natural inclination of young women drawn as they were to nursing, to be creatures with a kind disposition and intent on bringing hope and happiness to the lives of hospitalised children. At the same time these nurses accepted for themselves a code of behaviour that was professional in its orientation and put the welfare of the child before their own.

1919–1959: Science and professionalism, faltering care

Nursing has never been independent of wider society. The period between 1852 and 1920 was heavily influenced by Victorian romanticism, the strength of the Christian church and by a new awakening that society possessed a responsibility to care for the weak. British society around World War I subsequently began to undergo change. World War I had demonstrated a lack of young men fit enough to go to battle, the notion of fixed social positions began to change and people were seen to be capable of improving themselves and climbing the social ladder. At the same time there began to be a new understanding of childhood that was behaviourist in its orientation (Watson 1928) and which complied with the way that 'science' was intruding into everyday life.

Science had already explained the origins of life itself (Darwin 1872) and it was considered that in time, science would provide all the answers to man's problems. Science would cure disease, organise nursing (Ashdown 1927) and tell us how to bring up our children (Hardyment 1995). In particular, child care was now seen as a scientific process; like behaviourism itself, our dealings with children would be objective, systematic and regularised. There would be one known way of managing children which if it worked for one child must be applied to all children. Children were no longer to be understood as individuals but as examples of a whole. In addition, behaviourism dictated that emotional and romantic notions of childhood were dangerously unscientific and therefore wrong. There was to be no room for emotionality; to the increasingly influential behaviourists, children simply did not possess social, emotional and psychological needs (see Watson 1928, Jolley 2007c).

There was a much higher degree of social conformity than is the case today. People were much more likely to follow orders, to respect their elders and 'betters' and to do what they were told. Government policy began to be applied more closely to people's everyday lives. More hospitals were built, more special schools. This was the age of the scout movement and where military uniformity complied so well with scientific notions of objective and systematic approaches. It should not then surprise you that this was also the age of the eugenics movement (Galton 1905) which aimed to purify the Anglo-Saxon race at the expense of children less worthy in colour, handicap and breeding. Of course the Nazis took eugenics to its horrific conclusion but the degree to which eugenic principles were influential in this country should not be underestimated (see Welshman 1997).

Children's nursing became a 'harder' discipline that largely excluded parents from the care of the hospitalised child (Jolley 2007c). The Nurses Act of 1919 gave children's nurses the status of State Registration (Lindsay 2001). Nurses began to see themselves as 'professionals' and if not scientists themselves they worked intimately with Medicine which was, of course, 'science'. This effectively alienated them from parents who were seen as emotional and uneducated. Parents were often blamed for causing the child's illness by providing an inadequate diet and insufficient fresh air. Parents, especially mothers, were considered too emotional and therefore unable to provide the care needed by the child (Jolley 2004).

The most well understood effect of this period is the way in which parents were able to visit their child in hospital only for perhaps half an hour a week and in some cases not at all. Once children were separated from their parents in this way, they would initially cry but would eventually *'settle in'*, meaning that they would become quieter and more compliant. So it was that wards were full of bed-ridden children, separated from their families often for months at a time. Jolley (2004) provides some accounts from now-elderly people looking back on what it was like to be a child in hospital during this period. Some of the children's stories from this period are quite harrowing but they provide an important lesson for us today:

> If you want me to actually choose one thing, I think it was the powerlessness. I wasn't anything. I had no-one on my side to protect me, I was just there to be done to. Yes, I think that was it, the powerlessness ... So all I have thoughts on now is ... that they didn't really care. I think that they were getting on with their jobs. The fact that we were kids who (there must have been others who were as unhappy as I was). I don't think they cared a hoot what our feelings were, they were into bodies, not feelings ... I was completely and utterly isolated. It's like sticking a naked child in a pen with a load of farmyard chickens. You've got nothing to protect yourself with at all ... (p. 136).

Here, a nurse describes the way in which *science* did not actually involve thinking and problem solving but which instead was simply what existed in the literature of the day (Jolley 2004, p. 102):

> We went in to the theatre with them and then we brought them back into the anaesthetic room, we brought them round, then we took them back to the ward and we looked after them in the ward. That's how it was in the textbooks and we did it. You wouldn't deviate from that because it was what

worked fine and the patient was recovered as a result of it. So you know we never questioned how anything could be done differently because everything was right.

These nurses were not uncaring as they cared (Jolley 2006b). They took much pride in their work and it was especially rewarding when they were able to 'nurse a child better' (Jolley 2004). Nurses were clear about their contribution to the child's recovery and that their role was every bit as important, even more important than was that of the physician or surgeon (Jolley 2007b). Nor should it be considered that these nurses were ignorant of child psychology or of the child's social needs (Jolley 2007c). Nurses possessed the understanding of their day and this was essentially behaviourist. They were well educated and well trained, they did understand the science but the science was flawed. The truth, not understood at the time, is that children are individuals with individual needs for understanding, affection and love.

1959 to the present day: A refocus on CYP and family care

World War II brought significant changes to British society which was to have a direct impact on children's nursing. In time, parents would once again be welcomed into children's wards and would play an active part in their child's care. That care would also become more closely orientated to the CYP's needs as an individual and to the CYP's social and psychological needs.

World War II brought separation on a massive scale, not only though the armed conflict itself but through the mass evacuation of children from the towns and cities into the countryside (Titmuss 1950, Cleary *et al.* 1986, Macnicol 1986). This social exercise taught Britons everywhere that existing science and behaviourism did not provide a full explanation of children's needs as children. Instead it was clear that children did indeed have emotional needs, they needed their parents and their parents needed them. This was the love that is naturally present between parent and child and which behaviourism had ignored.

At the same time, war propaganda machine had told Britons that they were different from the German enemy because Britons were free and Britain was a democracy. The National Health Service, instituted in 1946, had put health care into the public domain. The hospitals now 'belonged' to the people. These changes empowered the British public to demand what they wanted from the National Health Service and for parents and carers, what they wanted was more access to their hospitalised sick children.

Research published by Bowlby and Robinson (Bowlby 1944a, b, Alsop-Shields and Mohay 2001) demonstrated that children needed their parents. Had it not been for World War II it is unlikely that nurses or the public would have taken notice of this research but it was instead exactly what they wanted to hear. The government was also keen to respond and published the Platt Report (Ministry of Health 1959) while at the same time the National Association for the Welfare of Children in Hospital (NAWCH) was formed to pressure hospitals to implement the Platt Report recommendations (Siddle 1991). The Platt Report recommended a move to what we would now call 'family-centred care'. This has been defined by Shields (Shields *et al.* 2006) as:

> … a way of caring for children and their families within health services which ensures that care is planned around the whole family, not just the individual child/person, and in which all the family members are recognized as care recipients (p. 1318).

This was a revolutionary change; children's nursing was still an inflexible organisation and it resisted the move to family-centred care (Duncombe 1979). Nevertheless social pressure, voiced largely through NAWCH, was unrelenting and inexorable. Today we can see the fruits of these labours in every children's ward in the land and in today's government policy (DH 2003, 2004) and in English law (DH 1989). Parents do not only visit their CYP every day, they often stay all day and all night too. Parents and other members of the CYP's family are not just 'visitors' but are active members of the care team and with whom children's nurses work compassionately, cooperatively and intimately.

Anne Casey's model of children's nursing (Casey 1988) illustrates this process well. Children's nursing has come to be a 'cooperation' of nursing, parenthood and childhood. Three essential elements in a professional activity designed to comfort and treat sick and injured children and to promote child health. In this model there is a new awareness, there is a new awareness of children that each child is an individual with individual needs and each an essential and inseparable part of a family.

Conclusion

Today, science and professionalism are both important aspects of children's nursing. However history has taught us that science is not static but that even though it is imperfect it continues to improve; nursing science today is characterised by a continuous struggle to discover better ways of delivering care. Professionalism too, has been redefined by history. It is now characterised by protecting the CYP in situations where other interests are legion and pressing and it is to accept the responsibility of making the profession better and more informed for children everywhere and for tomorrow.

Today there is room once again for Victorian romanticism (Jolley 2006c); CYP are important, childhood is important. Sick children deserve respect, protection and indeed affection. It is not possible to properly respect the individuality of a child without gaining a sense of affection for the human being that that endeavour reveals. So it is that children's nursing today employs ancient values, values that give the discipline depth and integrity. Indeed, it is not an exaggeration to say that it is such care as this, of the weakest and most defenceless members of society that defines civilisation itself (Jolley 2006b).

Further Reading

There are not many texts on nursing history; most modern historical studies are published in the nursing journals. For an informal introduction to children's nursing history you may wish to look at Jolley's series of short articles in Paediatric Nursing from 2006, some of which are referenced at the end of this chapter.

References

Alsop-Shields L and Mohay H (2001). John Bowlby and James Robertson: Theorists, scientists and crusaders for improvements in the care of children in hospital. *Journal of Advanced Nursing*, 35(1), 50–58.

Aries P (1962). *Centuries of Childhood*. London: Cape.

Armstrong G (1771). *An essay on the diseases most fatal to infants. To which are added rules to be observed in the nursing of sick children: With a particular view to those who are brought up by hand …/*. London: T. Cadell.

Armstrong G (1777). *An account of the diseases most incident to children, from their birth till the age of puberty; with a successful method of treating them. To which is added, an essay on nursing, also a general account of the Dispensary for the Infant Poor, from its first institution in 1769 to the present time*. London: T. Cadell.

Arton ME (1992). *The Development of Sick Children's Nursing, 1919–1939. History*. MPhil Thesis (unpublished), University of Bath.

Ashdown AM (1927). *A Complete System of Nursing*. London: Waverley Book Company Ltd.

Baly ME (1995). *Nursing and Social Change*. London: Routledge.

Bowers R (1999). *Thomas Phaer and the Boke of Chyldren*. London: Arizona State University.

Bowlby J (1944a). Forty-four juvenile thieves: Their characters and home life (I). *International Journal of Psychoanalysis*, 25, 19–53.

Bowlby J (1944b). Forty-four juvenile thieves: Their characters and home life (II). *International Journal of Psychoanalysis*, 25, 107–127.

Casey A (1988). A partnership with child and family. *Senior Nurse*, 8(4), 8–9.

Cleary J, Gray P, Rowlandson PH, Sainsbury CPQ and Davies MM (1986). Parental involvement in the lives of children in hospital. *Archives of Diseases in Childhood*, 61, 779–787.

Cunningham H (1995). *Children and Childhood in Western Society Since 1500*. London: Longman.

Darwin C (1872). *The Origin of the Species by Means of Natural Selection*. London: Murray.

DeMause L (1974). *The Evolution of Childhood. The History of Childhood: The Evolution of Parent Child Relationships as a Factor in History*. London: Souvenir Press.

Department of Health (DH) (1989). *Children Act 1989*. London: DH.

Department of Health (DH) (2003). *Getting the Right Start: National Service Framework for Children. Part I: Standard for Hospital Services*. London: DH.

Department of Health (DH) (2004). *Every Child Matters: Change for Children in Health Services*. London: DH.

Duncombe MA (1979). *A Brief History of the Association of British Paediatric Nurses, 1938–1975*. London: Association of British Paediatric Nurses.

Dunn PM (2006). Sir Denis Browne (1892–1927): The father of paediatric surgery in Britain. *Archives of Diseases in Childhood*, 89(Suppl 1), A54–A55.

Ellis H (2001). *A History of Surgery*. London: Greenwich Medical Media Limited.

Evans J (2004). Men nurses: A historical and feminist perspective. *Journal of Advanced Nursing*, 47(3), 321–328.

Forfar JO, Jackson ADM and Laurance BM (1989). *The British Paediatric Association, 1928–1988*. London: The Royal College of Child Health and Paediatrics.

Galton F (1905). *Eugenics, Its Definition, Scope and Aims*. London: Sociological Society of London.

Hardyment C (1995). *Perfect Parents: Baby Care Advice, Past and Present*. Oxford: Oxford University Press.

Jolley J (2004). *A Social History of Paediatric Nursing, 1920–1970. History*. PhD Thesis, University of Hull.

Jolley J (2006a). The first paediatrician. *Paediatric Nursing*, 18(7), 12.

Jolley J (2006b). The progress of care. *Paediatric Nursing*, 18(8), 12.

Jolley J (2006c). A mother's love. *Paediatric Nursing*, 18(5), 13.

Jolley J (2007a). Ahead of his time. *Paediatric Nursing*, 19(3), 12.

Jolley J (2007b). Lost causes and new hope. *Paediatric Nursing*, 19(2), 12.

Jolley J (2007c). Separation and psychological trauma: A paradox examined. *Paediatric Nursing*, 19(3), 22–25.

Lindsay B (2001). An atmosphere of recognition and respect? Sick children's nurses and medical men, 1880–1930. *International History of Nursing Journal*, 6(1), 4–9.

Mackintosh C (1997). A historical study of men in nursing. *Journal of Advanced Nursing*, 26(2), 232.

Macnicol J (1986). *The Evacuation of Schoolchildren. War and Social Change: British Society in the Second World War*, pp. 3–31. Manchester: H Smith.

Ministry of Health (1959). *The Report of the Committee on the Welfare of Children in Hospital (the Platt Report)*. HMSO, London.

Paget J (1874). Letter. *The Times*. London, p. 10.

Shields L, Pratt J and Hunter J (2006). Family centred care: A review of qualitative studies. *Journal of Clinical Nursing*, 15, 1317–1323.

Siddle J (1991). A voice for children NAWCH – the National Association for the Welfare of Children in Hospital. *British Journal of Theatre Nursing*, 1(6), 4–5.

Still GF (1931). *The History of Paediatrics: The Progress of the Study of Disease of Children Up to the End of the XVIIIth Century*. London: Royal College of Paediatrics and Child Health.

Titmuss R (1950). *Problems of Social Policy*. London: Longmans.

Wagner G (2004). *Thomas Coram, Gent, 1668–1751*. Woodbridge: Boydell Press.

Watson JB (1928). *Psychological Care of the Infant and Child*. London: Allen and Unwin.

Welshman J (1997). Eugenics and public health in Britain, 1900–40: Scenes from provincial life. *Urban History*, 24(1), 56–75.

West C (1854). *How to Nurse Sick Children*. London: Longman.

Wood C (1888). The training of nurses for sick children. *Nursing Record*, 1, 507–510.

Wyman AL (1984). The surgeoness: The female practitioner of surgery, 1400–1800. *Medical History*, 28, 22–41.

Yorkhill Hospitals Archive (1916–1932). Nurses Register 1916–1932. *YH8/1/4*, Glasgow.

Chapter 2
The Changing Educational Landscape of Children's and Young People's Nursing

Alan Glasper and Jim Richardson

The origins of education and registration for children's nurses

Twistington-Higgins (1952), in his book to commemorate the first hundred years of The Hospital for Sick Children, *Great Ormond Street Children's Hospital*, provides little detail on the education of children's nurses, but does articulate one of the founding aims of the hospital dated February 1852:

> To disseminate among all classes of the community but chiefly among the poor a better acquaintance with the management of infants and children during illness by employing it [The Hospital] as a school for the education of women in the special duties of children's nursing (p. 29).

This is the first record of a corporate strategy to train children's nurses, and was published some years before Nightingale set foot in the Crimea where she would make her name. Importantly, Twistington-Higgins asks 'what nurse could be expected to do as much for a sick and querulous child as his own mother?', perhaps recognising the skills necessary for this vocation. Yet his words are strangely at odds with Lindsay (2001), writing nearly 50 years later, who paints a somewhat black picture of the relationship between doctors and children's nurses. She asserts that a failure by nurses to capitalise on the early respect conferred on them is a root cause of their plight today.

Lindsay also believes that children's nurses may not have had the support they deserved from their general nurse colleagues in the aftermath of the 1919 Registration Act (Lindsay 2001). The apparent betrayal of this professional group, relegated initially to a supplementary register and therefore implicitly considered inferior to general nurses, is taken up by Price (1993), who describes general nurses' perceptions of children's nurses as being an anathema, semi-educated and prone to medical domination.

The fight for registration

At the time of the opening of The Hospital for Sick Children, nursing was still in the *Sairey Gamp* stage of educational development. Sairey Gamp, a major character in the Charles Dickens novel 'Martin Chuzzlewit' (1998), was vividly presented by the author as an untrained and disreputable 'nurse', both in the way she practised nursing and in her general demeanour as a woman who was invariably under the influence of alcohol! It can be argued, therefore, that the reason why the training of nurses figures so prominently in the original aims of the hospital is a recognition that specially trained children's nurses would be vital in enhancing the overall efficiency of care for sick children.

Although the informal training of sick children's nurses commenced immediately after the hospital opened in 1852, it was not until 1878 that the first formal training school was founded. Besser (1977), in his tribute to the 125 years of service of the Great Ormond Street Hospital, reminds the reader of Charles West's text book *How to Nurse Sick Children*. The book appeared in 1854, some 5 years before Nightingale's (1859) famous *Notes on Nursing*. Although Besser fails to mention the development of children's nursing, the publication of a book to illuminate the art of nursing sick children at a point in history when the future configuration of the profession was still unclear is remarkable. West's early commitment to the education of children's nurses was replicated through the development of other children's hospitals throughout Britain and further afield, in the decades following the opening of The Hospital for Sick Children, which Twistington-Higgins describes, quoting Dr West, 'as the mother of children's hospitals' (1952, p. 29).

Although the education of children's nurses was enshrined within the mission statements of many children's hospitals, the battle for statutory training and a professional recordable qualification was protracted and hard. On her return from the Crimea, Nightingale was a sick woman, suffering from what is now believed to be post-traumatic stress syndrome, but there is no doubt that she and her contemporaries such as Mary Seacole (http://medi-smart.com/history.htm) were determined to develop nursing. There is equally no doubt that Nightingale's preoccupation was with general nursing though in her *Notes* she states famously:

> Children: they are affected by the same things [as adults] but much more quickly and seriously (p. 72).

Additionally, there is evidence from the archives of Great Ormond Street Children's Hospital that West and Nightingale corresponded on the optimum way in which to nurse children. This is surprising, as Nightingale's knowledge of children, sick or well, was at best scanty. Yet the tendency of prominent people to seek advice about children from nurses who do not hold a children's nursing qualification continues to the present day. Arton (1992) reinforces this with descriptions of the matrons of the children's hospitals in the 1920s employing general nurses as paediatric ward sisters rather than registered sick children's nurses.

Ironically, it was Nightingale herself who was opposed to any such registration and effectively stifled its introduction until after her death. Baly (1980) describes how the Midwives Act passed in 1902, which mandated all midwives should undergo formal training and register with The Central Midwifes Board, made registration of general nurses an inevitability. Mrs Bedford Fenwick, the founder of the British Nurses Association, with over two decades of action to develop a nurses' register, continued to lobby even though private members' bills were withheld during the years of World War I hostilities. Conflict among the 'branches' of nursing was precipitated when the College of Nursing (later to become the Royal College of Nursing), a rival group to that of the British Nurses Association, but with the backing of the medical royal colleges, was founded in 1916. The College and the British Nurses Association decided that nurses who had only trained in a children's hospital should not be included on the proposed register of nurses. Furthermore, no attempt was made to include children's nurses on the proposed supplementary register which was to include only male nurses, mental nurses and fever nurses.

It is hardly surprising, therefore, that the children's hospitals, in receiving little or no support from the nurses' organisations, decided to take unilateral action. Glasper (1995) reports that this lack of support from senior general nurses caused great consternation among the children's hospitals throughout the UK. It was actually a group of children's hospitals in London, led by The Hospital for Sick Children, which sent a petition to the Privy Council opposing the petition sent by the British Nurses Association for a supplementary register that did not include children's nurses. Interestingly the senior physician at The Hospital for Sick Children, Arthur Francis Voelcker is most eloquent and persuasive in the petition stating that:

> The Empire will suffer because the saving of young life and the rearing of healthy children are becoming of increasing importance to our national welfare. If the numerous efforts to save infant life and to secure a healthy race are to be effective it is essential that Nurses should be specially trained in the nursing and care of sick children and that there should be an adequate supply of persons so trained and that their status as Children's Nurses should be fully recognised (Great Ormond Street Archive 1917).

Such stirring words were meant to reinforce the commitment of the children's hospitals in protecting their interests. Perhaps the greatest coup of The Hospital for Sick Children was in enrolling the Princess Royal as a probationer in 1918 during the period of negotiations related to the registration issue. The Princess Royal's status as a probationer children's nurse would have undoubtedly helped in allowing the children's hospitals make a better case for professionalism. Miles (1986, part 2) points out that children's nursing in the wake of the Princess Royal became eminently respectable and furthermore an ideal preparation for marriage and motherhood. Royal patronage of Great Ormond Street Children's Hospital continues to the present day.

There was intense debate surrounding the development of a supplementary register for sick children's nurses (Barlow and Swanwick 1994), and Arton (1987, 1988) provides a fascinating insight into the internecine warfare waged by the differing camps. Victory was finally achieved in December 1919 when the Nurses Bill received royal assent, with a mandate to create a General Nursing Council for England and Wales, Scotland and Northern Ireland. In addition to the general part of the register, a number of supplementary parts including the names of nurses trained in the nursing of sick children were included.

Arton (1988) reports that the main opposers of the inclusion of sick children's nurses to the register, led by Bedford Fenwick, believed such registers would be short lived. Since then, and after 82 years of its existence, the longevity of the children's nursing profession would seem to be assured. However upon closer examination, the progress of the register for such nurses can be seen to be fraught with difficulties. Great Ormond Street Children's Hospital most famous matron, Catherine Jane Wood, has left children's nurses a powerful legacy, as it was she who first stated that 'Sick Children require special nursing and sick children's nurses require special training' (Wood 1888). Of the initial 119 ladies who registered as children's nurses on the first published register in 1922, no less than 27 trained at the Hospital for Sick Children, Great Ormond Street (UKCC/NMC Archives Personal Correspondence).

The sick children's nursing register (part 8) lived on until the publication of Project 2000 in the late 1980s but not as a direct entry course (apart from in Scotland). Prejudice against a single RSCN qualification led many children's nurses to undertake further training as a registered general nurse to enable them to secure promotion to sister/charge nurse grade. The direct entry course was gradually phased out in England in the early 1960s (1970s in Northern Ireland, Wales never offered a course) and was replaced by a combined course spread over 3 years and 8 months which combined the sick children's training with general training. The numbers trained were small and the course was offered by only a few of the large children's hospitals. The majority of the trained children's nurses were subsequently trained via the expensive post-qualifying route which is now almost extinct because of cuts in commissions.

The introduction of the Project 2000 preregistration nurse education programmes resurrected the direct entry route to children's nursing, and since then applications to UK universities have been buoyant.

Contemporary children's nursing

The publication of the National Service Frameworks (NSF) for Children, Young People and Maternity Services (DH 2004c, WAG 2005) and their counterparts in Scotland and Northern Ireland reinforce the importance of a workforce that is committed to delivering the high standards that children/young people and their parents/guardians deserve in society. This is particularly important when children and young people (CYP) are ill. One of the stated principles for hospital services in the NSF for Children (NSF 2004) is that CYP should receive appropriate high quality evidence-based care delivered by staff who have the appropriate knowledge and skills.

It is the view, however, of some senior practitioners, articulated through the Association of Chief Children's Nurses, that contemporary CYP nurses in training may lack the skills necessary to meet the aspirations of contemporary policies such as those communicated in the NSF. Furthermore, the predicted demand for health care professionals such as CYP nurses far outstrips the projected supply.

In March 2005 members of the Nursing and Midwifery Council (NMC) considered concerns about the fitness for practice of some registrants at the point of registration. The Council has obligations under the Nursing and Midwifery Order 2001, and articles 21 and 22 relate directly to establishing and keeping under review standards for fitness to practise, competence and lack of competence. The Council has established a Coalition of senior stakeholders chaired by the President of the NMC to inform the discussion, and it also set up two *Task and Finish* Groups which included key stakeholders from all four UK countries. These groups have examined how fitness for practice could be better assured at the point of registration, and what support might be afforded to new registrants. Some areas discussed by the Coalition have included:

- Importance of stakeholder partnerships.
- Student selection.
- Requirements for literacy and numeracy.
- UK-wide standards of competence.
- Need for thorough skills rehearsal and testing.
- Need for mentors to have sufficient time to make judgements.
- Benefits of practice facilitators providing student and mentor support.
- Meeting the challenges of high student numbers requiring practice placements.
- Longer placements.
- Support in the post-qualifying period.

Additionally, the NMC is mandated under the auspices of the now defunct UKCC (the United Kingdom Central Council for Nursing, Midwifery and Health Visiting), through its Post Commission Development Group, to consider among others its recommendations for the future of the now preregistration fields of practice (formerly branches) (UKCC 2001). These are:

1. The current structure enhanced with practice experience divided equally between hospital and community settings.
2. The four current branches integrated with social care.

3. Six branches of nursing, including new separate branches of nursing for older people and community setting.
4. Two branches of nursing, child and adult.
5. Two branches of nursing, hospital and community.
6. The generalist nurse with specialisation following registration.

Furthermore, it is within the key area of skills and knowledge that some criticisms have been levelled at newly qualified CYP nurses and the academics who prepare them (UKCC 1999). There is therefore a perception among some senior nurse practitioners that student nurses at the point of registration do not have the acute care skills necessary for contemporary practice within the acute care sector. It is noteworthy that these perceptions have not been substantiated through a rigorous evaluation process. This means that such perceptions remain at the level of anecdote. The crux of this argument relates to the dilemma facing curriculum developers in deciding whether to adopt generalist or specialist modules and placements. Casey *et al.* (2001) have endeavoured to delineate the contribution of the so-called generalist CYP nurses and specialist CYP nurses. They believe that CYP nursing roles need to be fully dissected and explored to determine with considerable accuracy the skills and competencies, which are commensurate with the terms 'generalist nurse' and 'specialist nurse'.

This dilemma is confounded by one of the frequent complaints levelled at nurse educators, which is that there is a gap between theory and practice. There is a plethora of literature about the theory–practice gap and the term is often used as a derogatory expression to explain a skill deficit in a student or recently qualified staff nurse. In essence, the theory–practice gap is the distance between what is actually taught in a university classroom, and what really happens in clinical practice. Corlett (2000) has identified that the perception of students is that the gap is huge whereas nurse teachers perceive it to be small.

Similarly, Doman and Browning (2001) believe it to be over exaggerated, suggesting that regular and sustained collaboration between educators and clinicians is the key to a successful curriculum, a curriculum in which 'real world nursing' holds sway. However, Landers (2000) believes that the clinical environment and therefore the skills to navigate it are constantly changing, leading inevitably to discrepancies between what is taught and what is delivered at the bedside. The views of students about the theory–practice gap have been explored by Hislop *et al.* (1996) who argue that the arrival of the heralded *knowledgeable doer* will only come about when the phasing of university course work is carefully orientated with student placement allocation to promote the integration of theory with practice.

Additionally, perennial shortages of CYP nurses have been reported since the Court Committee revealed its findings in 1976, and Cox *et al.* (2003) have also indicated that the influence of course experiences is important to the future career plans of CYP nurses and the areas where they will choose to work. Although it is recognised that registration to the now part 1 (child field of practice) of the NMC register is somewhat different to that which governed entry to part 8, senior nurses in clinical practice still want all the attributes of the old register whose very title *Registered Sick Children's Nurse* conveyed the acute care focus expected of this group of nurses.

Clearly the acquisition of clinical skills remains a primary focus of children's nursing. The introduction of the new Project 2000 UKCC (now NMC) register in 1988 heralded the emergence of the registered nurse (child) whose curriculum was significantly different from that of the previous model. This new curriculum, which is still the basis of current education practice, reflected the health of CYP in society as whole rather than sick children in acute care settings. Casey *et al.* (2001) use the notion of the generalist children's nurse and articulate the various areas in which newly registered CYP nurses may work. The CYP post-millennium nurse, therefore, needs a different type of education if they are to work in the diverse areas where children may be nursed. This can range from a school setting to an acute hospital setting, so the types of client exposure necessary to meet the programme outcomes are likely to be eclectic. However, the very broadness of programmes in which students are given placements in non-acute areas may not fit the expected acute care profiles which the majority of applicants and employers currently look for.

Since the publication of *Fitness for Practice* (UKCC 1999), most preregistration nursing curricula embrace the principles of enquiry-based learning (EBL) as a method of educating students. EBL uses genuine real life client scenarios which provide students with an opportunity to explore a range of issues pertaining directly to client care in a variety of contemporary nursing settings (Glasper 2001). Despite this, Clark and Davies (2004) highlight the difficulty in ensuring sufficient clinical learning opportunities for child branch students, and reflect the voice of their own students who articulate their lack of confidence in relation to child specific clinical skills. Nevertheless, Price (2002), writing 2 years earlier, points out that only 3% of nursing students leave their programme because of dissatisfaction with the course or the practice elements.

This does not imply that all student nurses are necessarily happy with their course or its content. Glasper *et al.* (2006) have identified a number of areas where student dissatisfaction with their course is manifest. In this study, students in three universities surveyed identified the issue of under-capacity of student clinical placements as being within their top five items hindering personal progress. This leads to a situation where there are too many students allocated to a particular clinical area which in turn stretches the ability of mentors to offer an equitable service to all.

Meerabeau (2001) argues that the role of the educational commissioners had an unprecedented effect on the entire direction of nursing education within the independent universities, and highlights that there has been considerable debate on whether the educational reforms to nursing have actually produced nurses with the appropriate skills necessary for their purpose. The future relationship between those who commission nursing programmes and Higher Education Institutions (HEI) will therefore be based on an equitable resolution of the perennial clinical placement capacity crisis which bedevils some universities. This might be exacerbated as the necessity for sign-off mentors to be on the same part of the register as the students they were supervising came into force in October 2007.

Preregistration CYP nursing

Concerns about the health care curriculum and training are not unique to nursing. Richardson *et al.* (2006) used a SWOT analysis to consider preregistration children's nursing in the UK. From a sample of 13 universities they were able to show a number of strengths to the existing preparation including the continued success of the child branch since its reintroduction in 1988, and buoyant recruitment with an average of eight applicants per available university place. The availability of direct entry into the child field of practice is in keeping with the recommendation of numerous policy drivers such as the NSF.

The current curriculum has been designed to prepare CYP nurses to care for children from prematurity through to young adulthood. The diversity of experiences offered to students throughout their training which includes acute care, enduring health needs (chronicity, disability), mental health, learning disabilities, and high dependency care is perceived as fulfilling the vision of the NSF in providing high quality care for CYP wherever and whenever required. The introduction into the curriculum of EBL, for example, in which real life examples of child care scenarios are used, is providing CYP nurses with opportunities of exploring a range of issues directly pertaining to care in a variety of settings (Glasper 2001). Additionally, the utilisation of practical modules, where a greater emphasis is placed on skills teaching, is recognised as being particularly helpful in allowing students to hone and practice their skills before entering new clinical environments.

Nevertheless Richardson *et al.* (2006) also revealed a number of weaknesses to current methods of preparing CYP nurses. These include an affirmation of Meerabeau's (2001) findings which highlight the perceptions of some students that the nursing curriculum is adult and physical health orientated although the NMC themselves advocate branch specificity from day one of the nursing programmes. The most strident of those aspects of the weaknesses of the current system of educating CYP nurses is the limited capacity of placement circuits to meet commissioned student numbers. The current European Union requirements stipulate that student nurses have to complete 2300 hours of practice time in direct contact with patients.

The NMC is still considering proposals which might allow student nurses to gain some of their practice hours, especially in relation to skills acquisition, in skills laboratories. Clarke *et al.* (2003) believe that it is the quality of clinical placements which has the most noteworthy impact on how students learn in practice, and this will need to be reflected in any future change to practice hours. There remain concerns that there are too few acute care experiences, often at an inadequate level, for child branch students which may lead potentially to skills deficits among student groups.

Clifford (1999) believes it is critical that nurse educators retain the capacity to support education at the interface between theory and practice. She postulates further that this is what gives nurse educators their unique position in the higher education sector. Despite this, many nurse educators and clinicians look back to the days when all nurse teachers were part of the NHS workforce, and clinical teachers acted as a conduit between the student, the school and the clinical environment. Furthermore Richardson *et al.* (2006) report that academics have identified that lecturer support to individual students has deteriorated as commissions for larger student groups grows year on year. In developing the role of the CYP nurse there is clearly an opportunity in the light of the NSF to further develop and focus their work.

Crucially, if the government's modernisation agenda for health and social care to put the patient and carer at the forefront is to become a reality, then artificial demarcations within the current workforce have to be eroded. In light of the profound changes anticipated in health and social care roles, Humphris and Hean (2004) believe that this creates opportunities for health care professionals to work together for the benefit of patients and their carers. Richardson *et al.* (2006) also highlight the primary threat to the profession, that is a change in the professional register. Much has been written about the generic nurse; and CYP academics and practitioners remain concerned of any review by the NMC, in terms of its potential to threaten intrinsically, the long-term survival of their part of the profession.

Post-qualifying CYP nursing

The provision of pre- and post-registration CYP nurse education is inextricably linked, and from an analysis of data from 17 UK universities, Ellis *et al.* (2007) have offered a number of strengths and weaknesses to the existing UK provision. When the Department of Health (DH) rolled out its plans for modernising the pay structure of all health care professionals, Agenda for Change (DH 2004a) and its related pay spines became closely linked to the NHS Knowledge and Skills Framework (KSF) (DH 2004b). The latter provides a way of recognising the skills and knowledge that a nurse needs to apply to be effective in a particular NHS post. The KSF should ensure that better links exist between education, development and career, and pay progression, thus making post-registration training and education pivotal to the whole process.

The once robust system of kite marking post-qualifying courses has not yet been replaced by the NMC, who are still reviewing their stance on post-registration education of nurses. Although some specialist practice qualifications are still recordable by the NMC (such as Nurse Teacher preparation), and these courses are conjointly approved by them and the individual HEI, most courses are now developed and approved solely by the HEI concerned.

In 2006 the chief nursing officer of England, Christine Beasley, on behalf of all the countries of the UK launched an initiative which aims to give direction to a modernisation of the nursing profession (DH 2006) based on post-registration career pathways. Although the context of nursing is changing for all fields of practice, the challenges for CYP nurses are immense, with shorter hospital stays, rising levels of acuity and the emergence of new diseases such as type 2 diabetes linked to childhood obesity. Additionally, health inequalities linked to high levels of teenage pregnancy impact infant mortality rates which vary from one geographical area of the country to another.

Such changes to care demand link to advances in treatment and treatment technology which require nurses who are fit for practice across the spectrum of CYP care. It can be argued that the care sick children receive is only ever as good as the CYP nurses who deliver it. This places education, training and development of CYP nurses at the forefront of care delivery. Although the KSF provides a sound structure for the future direction of CYP nursing, it will be the responsibility of the profession to interpret generic competencies embedded within KSF to develop a post-registration career pathway which meets the aspirations of practitioners, managers and educationalists as they proactively plan the workforce of the future.

CYP nurses are familiar with partnership, working both with fellow professionals from within and without the health care team and with families and children. This places them in a strong leadership role for the other fields of practice that may not have the same depth of intra-agency experience as that of CYP nurses. Tomorrow's CYP nurse will need to work flexibly across health care boundaries, and have advanced skills to care for children with complex needs in acute and chronic settings. Gaining these multifaceted skills, knowledge and attitudes will require a level of unprecedented partnership between educators and commissioners to assure that the future provision of care is commensurate with the health needs of children, young people and their families.

One area of knowledge which has often come under scrutiny is a working understanding of human biology, which many practitioners believe to be fundamental to care delivery. Work with staff nurses (Clancy *et al.* 2000) has shown that they are not strongly confident of their biological knowledge base within their field of practice, or their ability to articulate this knowledge to patients. Although the mission of the NMC has been on the maintenance and improvement of professional knowledge and competence, Furze and Pearcey (1999) believe that there are barriers to post-registration education, not the least a lack of available places and funding. Importantly they also raise the spectre of the lack of an evidence base to underpin the efficacy of post-registration nurse education, crucial in a cash strapped NHS. In addition Jordan (2000), in exploring the gap between the post-registration educational input of nurses and the care that patients receive, argues that the curriculum itself should be evidence based and orientated to the needs of clinical roles over scholarly career aspirations of individuals or academic departments.

It is the need to provide to commissioners the evidence of the impact of post-registration education which should motivate those responsible for the design and implementation of programmes within nursing. Burchell *et al.* (2002) have addressed this in a case study of school teachers undertaking post-qualifying education, where there was an expectation that such education would make a difference in the classroom. They conclude that post-qualifying educational outcomes which are targeted at maintaining the motivation of the recipient and their professional values will make a difference in the workplace. It is this need to make a difference in the workplace of nursing which has led Tennant and Field (2004) to formally evaluate a post-registration intensive care course. Through a small study ($n = 10$) they were able to show that the nurses undertaking it had a subsequent positive impact on practice.

In their analysis of post-registration education of CYP nurses, Ellis *et al.* (2007) have given a unique insight into the national perception of academics in the current landscape of post-registration education. The primary strength of the existing provision is that it is linked to an inter-professional framework, which promotes evidence-based practice. Despite unsubstantiated criticisms about theory–practice links, Ellis *et al.* (2007) assert that post-registration courses are taught by people who are clinically credible.

A major strength of current post-registration education is flexibility of provision. This ensures that the workforce is supported especially with regard to acquiring the skills knowledge and attitudes demanded by Agenda for Change (DH 2004a) banding and KSF (DH 2004b). This is particularly evident in the growth of work-based modules which actually allow registrants seeking to increase their skills to themselves earn and learn without financially penalising their employers. Crucially it is believed that post-registration education is linked to the acquisition and development of advanced practice skills which in turn enhances career prospects because of the direct link to the KSF and ultimately grade banding. Perhaps, in a world dominated by evidence-based health care, the CYP nursing workforce needs academic skills to function in an increasingly complex work environment. To operate at this level, nurses need the skills of critical appraisal and analysis if they are to fully comprehend and utilise research findings within their area of practice. Post-registration opportunities can provide this element of knowledge transfer.

Ellis *et al.* (2007) also reveal some weaknesses, such as the small number of potential post-registration students. The CYP field of practice is but a small percentage of the 650,000 plus nursing workforce in the UK (NMC 2003), and consequently, the numbers of potential post-registration students available to undertake courses is less than optimum. Perhaps because of this small pool of potential students, post-registration courses for CYP nurses are not CYP specific, and there may therefore be insufficient child and young person specific courses available to registrants.

This situation is exacerbated by the limited numbers of students being released from practice for further study. Chambers (2007) reflects this in highlighting the diminished support practice areas are able to give to the professional development of their nurses, and in revealing the stark reality that many who are fortunate enough to gain a place on a post-registration course frequently find themselves being unable to attend because of staff shortages, exacerbated by job freezes or having to make significant sacrifices both in terms of time and money. On the other hand, alternative models of delivery of post-registration education such as e-learning and work-based learning have great potential in this climate.

The growth and interest in inter-professional courses beyond primary registration represents a major opportunity for a small field of practice such as CYP nursing, and the NSF (DH 2003, WAG 2004) stress the importance of professionals working together for the overall benefit of the children and families they care for. In reflecting on the changing role of nurses, the need for staff to undertake further post-qualifying education is inevitably bound to the KSF and Agenda for Change (DH 2004a). Only in reconciling the design of new courses with the expectations of managers regarding the competencies necessary for certain roles, academics will be able to link their courses fundamentally to the career and professional development aspirations of their future potential students.

This will also help integrate the growth in the Masters and taught doctorate programmes for senior nurses aspiring to differing roles. Despite this, Ellis *et al.* (2007) suggest that many universities are consolidating and amalgamating their portfolio of post-registration courses in light of changing funding streams. In real terms this has led to a reduction in the number of courses available to CYP nurses, and when coupled with financial cuts within NHS organisations and insufficient resources the result is a lower numbers of potential students.

The views of students

The CYP nursing students are the life blood of the profession, and their views of their own education are important to educators in their challenge to write curricula of the future. Glasper *et al.* (2006) have examined the world of learning through an analysis of student perceptions of their preparation. The factors which helped students most in their quest to become CYP nurses included the delivery of specialist lectures from child branch nurse lecturers, having good clinical placements with mentors who want to support students, and having the support of friends and family. Perhaps the most important factor was the desire to become a good CYP nurse, and wanting to work with children. The factors which hindered students included having unsupportive mentors who misjudge student abilities, lack of academic resources including library reading materials, too many students in each clinical area, and understaffing on wards, leading to a reliance on students to provide unsupervised care.

Writing in 2002, child branch student Wendy Horseman (2002) laments the lack of interest shown to her by her mentor during a placement. She reported that no less than 5 of her fellow students from a cohort of 16 experienced similar unpleasantnesses during placements. She concludes by suggesting that poor supervision may be directly linked to increased student attrition from child branch courses.

With a paucity of research evidence to underpin the value of children's nursing, have articulated the need for further exploration of just what qualities, both personal and practical, are needed by individuals seeking to become CYP nurses. Evans (2001) has indicated that towards the end of their education students are concerned about acquiring the skills of a staff nurse. The complex world of clinical practice and the transition from student, to staff nurse, to mentor happens quickly. It is therefore crucial that mentors should be committed and highly motivated individuals. These attributes are essential if mentors are to be role models for the future registered members of the profession. Doman and Browning (2001) articulate other qualities such as mutual respect and trust, coupled with excellence in communication skills, as being essential in fostering collaboration between education and practice.

Glasper *et al.* (2006) have shown that students appreciate good tutorial support and having theory being constantly illuminated with examples from practice. Field of practice identity and the acquisition of those attributes which make up the character of the CYP nurse remain of vital importance, and necessitates vigilance in ensuring that students continue to acquire the necessary skills, knowledge and attitudes appropriate to the art and science of their profession.

The issue of under-capacity of clinical placements has been identified by Glasper *et al.* (2006) as being capable of hindering student progress. This leads to a situation where there are too many students allocated to a particular clinical area which in turn stretches the ability of mentors to offer an equitable service to all. A finding in a Mori poll reported in the Guardian (Carvel 2003) reported that a third of surveyed students had been abandoned by their mentor and left in sole charge of patients. The absolute key to the future of nurse education is the constructive and productive relationship between teacher, student and clinical mentor. Today's contemporary student is tomorrow's clinical mentor, and that mentor will be the net recipient of what was learned and observed during the formative student years.

The lack of collaboration between the clinical areas and educational institutions has been described by Corlett (2000), who vehemently laments the lack of clarity related to link teacher roles. The link teacher may be the key to bridging the gaps between the student and clinical mentor and perhaps this role requires strengthening.

Comment and conclusions

Reflecting on the education of CYP nurses, it is apparent that there are three players whose needs must be considered in order to make pre- and post-registration education successful. The individual students require education that provides them with academic accreditation, will be recognised as valuable, will benefit their career progression, and is motivating, achievable and affordable. The service provider is interested in education that will add quality/skill to the individual's performance. The university wants to provide quality education that is academically recognised, clinically credible, valued by the student, cost-effective and valued by the university. All these courses will also need to be evidence based, linked to the KSF, are CYP specific and taught by lecturers who are academically and clinically credible.

References

Arton ME (1987). The caretaker General Nursing Council and Sick Children's Nursing 1920–1923. *RCN History of Nursing Bulletin*, 2(1), 1–7.

Arton ME (1988). The supplementary register for sick children's nurses – accident or design. *RCN History of Nursing Bulletin*, 2(4), 24–28.

Arton ME (1992). *Development of Sick Children's Nursing 1919–1939*. MPhil Thesis (unpublished), University of Bath.

Baly ME (1980). *Nursing and Social Change*, 2nd edn. London: Routledge, Taylor and Francis.

Barlow S and Swanwick M (1994). Supplementary benefits. *Paediatric Nursing*, 6(3), 16–17.

Besser FS (1997). Great Ormond Street anniversary. *Nursing Mirror*, 144(6), 60–63.

Burchell H, Dyson J and Rees M (2002). Making a difference: A study of the impact of continuing professional development on professional practice. *Journal of In-Service Education*, 28(2), 219–229.

Carvel J (2003). Patients left in care of trainee nurses. *The Guardian (Editorial)*, 28 April.

Casey A, Gibson F and Hooker L (2001). Role development in children's nursing: Dimensions terminology and practice framework. *Paediatric Nursing*, 13(2), 36–40.

Chambers D (2007). Is the modern NHS fit for nursing students? *British Journal of Nursing*, 16(2), 74–75.

Clancy J, McVicar A and Bird D (2000). Getting it right? An exploration of issues relating to the biological sciences in nurse education and nursing practice. *Journal of Advanced Nursing*, 32(6), 1522–1532.

Clark D and Davies J (2004). Clinical skills acquisition in children's nursing: An international perspective. *Paediatric Nursing*, 16(2), 23–26.

Clarke CL, Gibb CE and Ramprogus V (2003). Clinical learning environments: An evaluation of an innovative role to support pre-registration nursing placements. *Learning in Health and Social Care*, 2(2), 105–115.

Clifford C (1999). The clinical role of the nurse teacher: A conceptual framework. *Journal of Advanced Nursing*, 30(1), 179–185.

Corlett J (2000). The perceptions of nurse teachers, student nurses and preceptors of the theory–practice gap in nurse education. *Nurse Education Today*, 20, 499–505.

Cox S, Murrells T and Robinson S (2003). Careers in child health nursing: The influence of course experiences. *Paediatric Nursing*, 15(10), 36–41.

Dickens C (1998) *Martin Chuzzlewitt*, Oxford. Oxford World Classics, Oxford University Press.

Department of Health (DH) (2003). *National Service Framework for Children Standard for Hospital Service*. London: DH.

Department of Health (DH) (2004a). *Agenda for Change: Final Agreement*. London: DH.

Department of Health (DH) (2004b). *The NHS Knowledge and Skills Framework (NHS KSF) and the Development Review Process*. London: DH.

Department of Health (DH) (2004c). *National Service Framework for Children, Young People and Maternity Services*. London: DH.

Department of Health (DH) (2006). *Modernising Nursing Careers: Setting the Direction*. London: DH.

Doman M and Browning R (2001). Gap? What gap? Celebrating collaboration between education and practice. *Paediatric Nursing*, 13(9), 34–37.

Ellis J, Glasper EA, McEwing G and Richardson J (2007). *The future of post-registration education for children's and young people's nursing: A SWOT analysis. Journal of Children's and Young People's Nursing*, 1(2), 64–71.

Evans K (2001). Expectations of newly qualified nurses. *Nursing Standard*, 15(410), 33–38.

Furze G and Pearcey P (1999). Continuing education in nursing: A review of the literature. *Journal of Advanced Nursing*, 29(92), 355–363.

Glasper EA (1995). The value of children's nursing in the third millennium. *British Journal of Nursing*, 4(1), 27–30.

Glasper EA (2001). Child health nurses' perceptions of enquiry-based learning. *British Journal of Nursing*, 10(20), 1343–1349.

Glasper EA, Richardson J and Whiting R (2006). The highs and lows of learning to be a children's nurse. *Paediatric Nursing*, 18(6), 22–26.

Great Ormond Street Archive (1917). *Petition in Opposition to the Petition for a Supplemental Charter by the Royal British Nurses' Association*. Presented 27 June 1917 to the King's Most Excellent Majesty in Council – presented by AF Voelcker, senior physician at the Hospital for Sick Children and Charles Edward Allan, member of the Committee of the Victoria Hospital for Children.

Hislop S, Inglis B, Cope P, Stoddart B and McIntosh C (1996). Situating theory in practice, student views of theory–practice in Project 2000 nursing programmes. *Journal of Advanced Nursing*, 23(1), 171–177.

Horseman W (2002). I want to be a nurse, but – a student's experience of clinical placements. *Paediatric Nursing*, 14(8), 34.

Humphris D and Hean S (2004). Educating the future workforce: Building the evidence about interprofessional learning. *Journal of Health Service Research Policy*, 9(1), 24–27.

Jordan S (2000). Educational input: Exploring the gap. *Journal of Advanced Nursing*, 31(20), 461–471.

Landers MG (2000). The theory–practice gap in nursing: The role of the nurse teacher. *Journal of Advanced Nursing*, 32(6), 1550–1556.

Lindsay B (2001). An atmosphere of recognition and respect? Sick children's nurses and medical men 1880–1930. *International History of Nursing Journal*, 6(1), 4–9.

Meerabeau E (2001). Back to the bedpans: The debate over pre-registration nursing education in England. *Journal of Advanced Nursing*, 34(4), 427–435.

Miles I (1986). The emergence of sick children's nursing. Part 2. *Nurse Education Today*, 6(3), 133–138.

Nightingale F (1859). *Notes on Nursing: What It Is and What It Is Not*. London: Duckworth and Company (1970 reprint).

NMC (2003). *NMC News*, December.

Price S (1993). Children's nursing: Lessons from the past. *Nursing Standard*, 7(50), 31–35.

Price S (2002). The recruitment and retention of children's nurses. *Paediatric Nursing*, 14(6), 39–43.

Richardson J, McEwing G and Glasper EA (2006). Pre-registration children's and young people's nurse preparation. A SWOT analysis. *Paediatric Nursing*, 18(10), 34–37.

Tennant S and Field R (2004). Continuing professional development: Does it make a difference? *Nursing in Critical Care*, 9(4), 167–172.

Twistington-Higgins T (1952). *Great Ormond Street 1852–1952*. Watford: Odhams Press Ltd.

United Kingdom Central Council for Nursing, Midwifery and Health Visiting (UKCC) (1999). *Fitness for Practice*. London: UKCC.

United Kingdom Central Council for Nursing, Midwifery and Health Visiting (UKCC) (2001). *Fitness for Practice and Purpose – The Report of the UKCC's Post Commission Development Group*. UKCC, London.

Welsh Assembly Government (WAG) (2005). *National Service Framework for Children, Young People and Maternity Services*. Cardiff: WAG.

Wood CJ (1888). The training of nurses for sick children. *The Nursing Record*, 6 December, 507–510.

Chapter 3

An International Comparison of Children's Nursing Roles

Anne Casey

Introduction

Making comparisons is useful for two reasons: to learn about others and to learn about ourselves. Understanding how other people or organisations approach the challenges that we face provides us with opportunities to confirm our own approaches or to consider changing the way we do things. It is for these reasons that the editors felt addition of a chapter comparing children's nursing roles in different countries would be useful.

In all countries, the social, political, economic and technological environments impact on health, health care and nursing (International Council of Nurses 2006). As these environments are constantly changing, it would not be sensible to provide tables of detailed differences between countries; the information would be out of date before the book goes to print. Instead, I have looked at how various factors have influenced the development of children's nursing roles with examples from different countries and health systems. These influences continue to have an impact on the evolution of all aspects of practice, from the type of care that nurses provide to their degree of autonomy in decision making. By the end of the chapter, you should have a good understanding of the factors that shape children's nursing roles as well as knowledge about specific differences between countries.

Figure 3.1 summarises these factors and is used as the organising framework for this chapter. You may find this model and others presented in the sections below useful for reviewing children's nursing roles in your practice setting or country, allowing you to see which factors might be altered to improve outcomes for children or to improve the lives and careers of children's nurses.

If you are planning to work as a children's nurse in a different country, the content of this chapter provides a framework for making sense of the context in which you will be working. The International Council of Nurses (ICN) (2002) has published a set of questions you should be asking, as follows: What are the requirements for registration, if any? The client population? The required competencies? The hierarchy of authority? Some of these issues are considered here, but specific guidance on working abroad is not covered; see Box 3.1 for useful sources of information about working abroad.

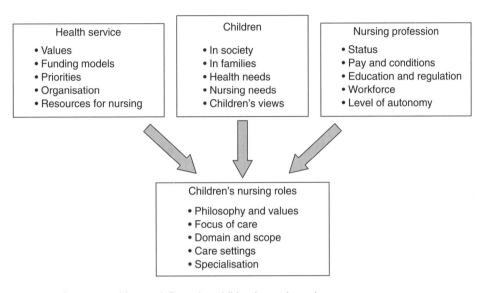

Fig. 3.1 Summary of factors influencing children's nursing roles.

Box 3.1   Working abroad: useful resources

Working as a nurse in...

Comprehensive general information from RCN Direct on line (RCN members only) with specific information on nursing in 62 countries from Australia to Zambia. www.rcn.org.uk/members/direct/ Tel: 0845 7726 100

Career moves and migration: critical questions

International Council of Nurses guidance including a list of questions you need to ask before deciding to work abroad. www.icn.ch/CareerMovesMigangl.pdf

Search for jobs abroad

Find useful tips and job opportunities or organisations in different countries on this site, which is part of NursingNetUK. www.nursingabroad.net/

Your questions answered

The information desk of the Royal College of Nursing International Office provides information for RCN members Tel: 020 7647 3610 or Email international.office@rcn.org.uk

Source material

Finding reliable sources of information on children's health needs, health services and nursing is challenging. Very general data are available from the World Health Organisation (WHO) and the United Nations Children's Fund (UNICEF) and on the websites of national health departments. But many countries including the UK do not have data, for example, on how many of their child citizens have disabilities or mental health problems and what services are provided for them. Systematic reviews and research reports provide useful snapshots of health needs and approaches to care, particularly reports of international studies, but many of these are in non-English language publications.

There are increasing numbers of reports of children and young people's views on their health needs both in professional literature and on websites designed to capture their input. The Internet is becoming an invaluable resource and is increasingly used to help children develop networks and exchange information with their peers, as well as providing professionals with insights into children's lives and health concerns (see UNICEF's Voices of Youth website, www.unicef.org/voy/, for an international example).

Data about nurses and nursing are poor in most countries. Few governments can provide information on how many nurses they educate and employ. Discovering the nature of nursing practice and roles is also challenging mainly because the obvious sources such as educational curricula and professional or governmental policy documents generally represent ideal views rather than reality. Here too, reviews and research reports are most helpful, particularly those that include an international dimension. Publications from the WHO and the ICN provided much of the material used in this chapter. It proved impossible to obtain reliable information about children's nursing in many countries, particularly in developing countries where the occasional article suggested educational courses were in place but nothing further was available. Box 3.2 provides a list of sources of what information can be obtained about children's health needs and children's nursing.

Definitions

Many countries use the United Nations (UN) definition of a child for legal purposes: 'every human being below the age of eighteen years unless, under the law applicable to the child, majority is attained earlier' (UN 1989, p. 2). However, health and social care organisations within and among countries differ widely in their policies for young people when treated as adults. For some there is no difference to begin with, but where a choice is possible, young people may be offered adult services at 12 years of age, others may remain in dedicated children's and young people's services until their early twenties.

When comparing countries, the questions that could be asked are as follows:

1. If there are specific children's services, up to what age are these provided?
2. How do children and young people see themselves in the health care system: do older children have a choice over whether their health needs are met in children's or adult services?

Box 3.2   Sources of Information about child health and children's nursing

'For every child ... health, education, equality, protection'

The UNICEF website and annual reports are the best source of information about progress of children's health and well-being across the globe. www.unicef.org

Health of children in Europe

The European Health Report 2005 summarises the major public health issues facing the region, particularly its children, and describing effective policy responses and providing data on health states in different countries. www.euro.who.int/ehr2005

Health of children and young people in the UK

National Statistics Online The Health of Children and Young People contains analysis of health and health-related behaviour among those aged under 20 years in the UK during the period 1990–2001. www.statistics.gov.uk/children/

Indicator of child health in English regions

The Association of Public Health Observatories (APHO) facilitates collaborative working of the Public Health Observatories (PHOs) and their equivalents in England, Wales, Scotland and Ireland. www.apho.org.uk/apho/viewResource.aspx?id=4492

Paediatric nursing in Europe

The website for the Paediatric Nursing Associations of Europe is hosted by the RCN and includes summaries of paediatric nursing in its member countries as well as position statements and meeting summaries. www2.rcn.org.uk/cyp/forums

---

Social, cultural and economic realities mean that childhood is experienced very differently in various countries and sectors of society. Even though childhood 'should be a separate space from adulthood, a time when children can grow and play, rest and learn' (UNICEF 2005, p. 43), in many countries children are forced to adopt adult roles prematurely and are then no longer viewed as children. The most important question for defining the subject of children's nursing care is how children are viewed and treated by their families and the society in which they live.

In many countries, nursing care of children will be carried out by nurses who are not qualified children's or paediatric nurses. Some places do not recognise such qualifications, and if they do, they may have a very different view of what a paediatric (or pediatric) nurse is and does. 'Children's nurse' is used in this chapter in its most general sense, meaning any nurse working with infants, children and young people. However, a qualified children's/paediatric nurse is

a nurse who has successfully completed a recognised course of study and practice experience in the nursing care of infants, children and adolescents/young people (Paediatric Nursing Associations of Europe 2005, p. 1).

Children's need for health care and nursing

Children's nurses' roles are first and foremost shaped by the health care needs of children (Fig. 3.1). These needs are not static, and although generalisations can be made about the health of children in different countries at particular points in time, it is important to remember that within countries children may be experiencing very different health problems, either because of their local situation or because they have recently arrived from another country. With immigration, global travel and variations in socioeconomic circumstances, big differences may be seen in health needs and how these are viewed by the child and the family living in the same street or town.

Patterns of disease

Mortality statistics illustrate these differences most profoundly: the under-five mortality rate in the least developed countries is 155 per 1000 live births; in industrialised countries, it is 6 (UNICEF 2005). Around 10.6 million children under the age of 5 die each year. According to the WHO Child Health Epidemiology Reference Group (Bryce *et al.* 2005), six causes account for 73% of these deaths: pneumonia, diarrhoea, malaria, neonatal pneumonia or sepsis, preterm delivery and asphyxia at birth. Undernutrition is an underlying cause of 53% of deaths in the under-fives (Bryce *et al.* 2005). Even in countries with relatively low child death rates, mortality statistics can demonstrate wide variations in health status.

For example, Robert *et al.* (2006) report that rates of death from injury and poisoning in children have fallen in England and Wales over the past 20 years, 'except for children in families in which no adult is in paid employment' (p?). European data on adolescents with cancer showed that 5-year survival for all cancers in 1988–1997 was 73% in Europe as a whole, with the major contribution of 57% in eastern Europe (Stiller *et al.* 2006). In some African countries, the gap in mortality between rich and poor children is smaller: the health services are limited even if you can afford them and the social conditions mean that diseases can spread more easily (UNICEF 2005).

Across Europe, there are large differences according to age, gender, geographical location and socioeconomic position both between and within countries (WHO Europe 2005). Eastern countries have higher morbidity and mortality among children suffering from respiratory and infectious diseases, injuries and poisoning, while disease patterns in western countries include more non-communicable disorders such as asthma, diabetes, obesity and mental health problems (WHO Europe 2005). In the UK, we see these kinds of differences in all kinds of child health statistics, for example, a UK-wide study of over 18,000 babies found higher rates of partial immunisation associated with living in ethnic or disadvantaged wards, larger families, one or teenaged parents, maternal smoking in pregnancy and admission to hospital by 9 months of age (Samad *et al.* 2006).

It is obvious that nursing roles will differ depending on the community that is being served, but health needs do not remain static. An important but under-researched area is the health problems children face in developing countries where old and emerging infectious diseases are still endemic but where incidence of chronic conditions and disability are rising with changing demographics, increased life expectancy and improvements in health care provision. While a country is in crisis or undeveloped, the health and nursing priorities are nutrition, immunisation and maternal health; as things start to improve, attention can be turned to other problems. In one example, a study of child injury in four developing countries (Ethiopia, Peru, Vietnam and India) found that maternal depression is a consistent risk factor across all the four countries and for all types of injury (Howe *et al.* 2006). As a country progresses, prevention strategies shift beyond clean water, food aid and immunisation; as infections are controlled, other conditions come to the fore and health services begin to develop paediatric subspecialties, with a need for nurses to be trained in those subspecialties (Wilimas *et al.* 2003).

Universal health needs

The UN Convention on the Rights of the Child (UN 1989) requires States to ensure that every child has access to 'the highest attainable standard of health and to facilities for the treatment of illness and rehabilitation of health' (Article 24.1). Children's rights include protection from all forms of harm, provision of adequate nutritious foods and clean drinking water, support for healthy development and education to improve life chances. Article 23 highlights specific rights for children with disabilities including access to 'education, training, health care services, rehabilitation services, preparation for employment and recreation opportunities' (UN 1989, Article 23.3). Translating these rights into needs that health and other services can respond to results in a list of high level interventions:

- Protection from abuse and other forms of physical, emotional and psychological harm.
- Promotion of good parenting, healthy lifestyles, growth, development, psychological and social well-being, independence and life opportunities.
- Prevention of disease and injury and their consequences.
- Early detection and management of illness, including mental illness and behavioural difficulties.
- Support for living with disability, chronic conditions and altered lives.
- Where death is inevitable, care and support to live with dying.

Most episodes of childhood illness will be managed by families without input from health care workers. In industrialised nations, children and young people are more frequent users of health care than adults. According to the Department of Health (2003), in England in a typical year, a pre-school child will see their general practitioner about six times, up to half of infants aged under 12 months and a quarter of older children will attend an emergency department. Even though they face different challenges to health and safety, all children and young people have the same basic needs and the same rights to health care. The ways that those needs are met in different parts of the world are compared in the next section.

Health care provision for children

Policy and values

Health care organisation and delivery differs depending on the underlying values of those who decide on health policy and allocate funding for services. According to Gillies (2003), the most common driver influencing health policy is finance, but political ideology will also have an impact. In the UK at least, high profile service failures have led to significant policy changes. Funding and prioritisation of children's services are significantly affected by how children are viewed in the society; even in countries that have ratified the UN convention, children may have low status and visibility and their health needs given lower priority. Girls may have lower status that boys and women who might otherwise advocate for children's services may not have the freedom to do so.

Factors that can be used to understand and compare health systems are found in policy publications and legislation from countries such as Canada, Australia and the UK. Gillies (2003) cites the values of the national health system embodied in the Canada Health Act, which includes accessibility, universality, comprehensiveness and public administration. The UK National Health Service (NHS) was founded on principles of comprehensive health care that was free at the point of delivery. Australia followed this model but has since moved towards a part publicly/part privately funded service, raising concerns about quality and equity of access (Gillies 2003).

Starfield and Shi (2002) studied the health systems in 13 industrialised countries to investigate links between policy and health. Five characteristics appeared to distinguish countries with children of overall good health from those with children of poor health at all ages:

1. Equitable distribution of resources.
2. Publicly accountable universal financial coverage.
3. Low cost sharing.
4. Comprehensive services.
5. Family-oriented services (Starfield and Shi 2002).

Many developed countries have recently adopted policy goals intended to shift health care delivery closer to the community, workplace and home, with less dependence on institutional care (WHO 1997). However, progress has been slow and is hampered by lack of resources, with continued focus on financing and structures, which 'tend to focus on acute hospitals and the role of doctors' (WHO

1997). This problem is well illustrated in current NHS policy aspirations that include more health promotion and care in the community, home and school. More emphasis has been placed on these subjects in nursing education, but the majority of children's nurses still work in acute care as there are few posts in primary and community care for qualified children's nurses.

Nurses' work and roles are shaped not so much by government policies themselves, but the outcome of their implementation, for example, the extent to which health care is largely located focuses on health promotion versus treatment for illness; is located in large hospitals versus community settings; and, most importantly, is based on the needs of children and young people versus the self-interest of professionals (Health Select Committee 1997). Equally important how children and families experience health care is the way in which values are shared by local health care teams with the children and their families. Shields and Nixon (2004) reporting on a study of values and attitudes to hospital care of children in Australia, England, Indonesia and Thailand concluded that although parents' and staff's expectations about delivery of care varied, basic concepts of family-centred care were similar.

In Finland, a study of nursing support for families during a child's illness illustrates the reality of values that are widely held but difficult to put into practice; both families and nurses suggested that better emotional and informational support related to time, more client-centred attitudes, the family being appreciated and listened to and more guidance at home (Sarajarvi *et al.* 2006). Sarajarvi and co-workers from their international literature review concluded that this problem of translating philosophies such as family-centred care into reality was common across the globe and that 'deeper consideration of possible underlying reasons for this phenomenon is called for' (p. 205).

Service models

There are a number of models that can help in understanding and comparing health service provision for children and young people. Models that combine the child's need with required infrastructure are the most useful: one of the simplest and most effective is the four-tier model of Child and Adolescent Mental Health Services (CAMHS) (Every Child Matters 2006). This sets out what kinds of professionals, with what skills, can most effectively and efficiently meet the differing levels of need of children and young people with mental health problems. A similar three-tier model has been adopted in Australia, although there are variations between states (Victorian Government 2006). In New Zealand, the first tier is not mentioned; CAMHS is described as a secondary service accepting referrals from other professionals, educational and community organisations although it is mainly community-based (Werry Centre 2006).

The diverse health care delivery systems in the US mean that the federal government has to be less directive, but it does provide guidance, education, media campaigns and advice on good practice for child and family mental health services. Implementation is left up to local communities under the 'systems of care' policy in which

> mental health, education, child welfare, juvenile justice, and other agencies work together to ensure that children with mental, emotional, and behavioural problems and their families have access to the services and supports they need to succeed (US Department of Health and Human Services 2006, http:// mentalhealth.samhsa.gov/cmhs/ChildrenCampaign/grantcomm.asp)

Similar wording is evident in most child health policies that you find on government websites: integrated, multi-agency working, centred on the child/young person and family and involving them in decision making and management.

Service design models such as the CAMHS tiers and the 'hub and spoke' model used to develop paediatric intensive care services in several countries demonstrate attempts to make effective use of expertise for the specialist care of relatively small numbers of children who may need to travel large distances for such services. They balance care 'close to home' with the need to centralise to maintain expertise and quality. They also define the roles and competencies of staff delivering the services at different points in the care pathway.

Care pathway or 'patient journey' models offer the best potential for establishing whether a service is really planned around the needs of the child. This approach is used to underpin health service policy for children in some countries and was used in the development of the national service frameworks in England and Wales. A number of exemplars of a child's journey through care were produced alongside the service frameworks and are being used to guide implementation including child with complex disability, asthma and autistic spectrum disorder and children requiring long-term ventilation in the community (Department for Education and Skills and Department of Health 2004).

These ideal pathways act as gold standards when undertaking comparisons; this is what a child and parent could expect in an equitable, well-managed health service mapped against the realities in their country or area within a country. The first part of any pathway, access to the health system, is perhaps the most important indicator as it highlights whether there are gaps and inequities in provision for children with different needs or circumstances.

Another useful tool for comparison is the various options for care that might be in place. How different countries manage transition for adolescents with chronic conditions or complex needs to adult services is a good example. According to the Department for Education and Skills and Department of Health (England) (2006):

> the most prevalent model for a transition service is not transition at all, but rather a transfer of young people to what looks like the most relevant adult clinic – or, worse still, discharge from the children's or young person's clinic with instructions to ask the GP for a referral to adult services (p. 25).

Their report lists possible models for transition:

- Follow-up service within the adult setting with no continuity from paediatric services.

- 'Seamless' clinic with both child and adult professionals providing ongoing care as appropriate.
- Life-long follow-up within the paediatric setting.
- Generic transition team within a children's hospital as is the case in one example from Canada.
- Generic transition co-ordinators for larger geographical regions as in an Australian example (Department for education and Skills and Department of Health 2006).

Children's views

Until recently the voices of children and young people were largely unheard in the health care arena. Gradually, the right of the child to be heard is being addressed mainly because of shifts in policy towards wider patient and public involvement in services and care. Comparing children's views of health, illness and health care could be the best way to assess the extent to which nurses in different countries are able to deliver child-centred, responsive services. Reports of children's views appear frequently in the literature, and guidance is widely available on involving children in decision making as well as in service planning and evaluation.

For example, Lindeke *et al.* (2006) interviewed 120 children on discharge from a tertiary centre in the US and found that pain and discomfort was the aspect of hospitalisation that needed most improvement. Children of all ages valued play activities and frequently described their positive relationships with hospital staff. An innovative study in England by six teenagers supported by a children's nurse researcher confirmed five health service quality factors from the child/young person's perspective (Moules 2004, p. 31). These were the following:

1. Good technical skills – 'nurses and doctors should take care to cause minimal pain, do things carefully, consider comfort and they must be well trained'.
2. Friendly staff – 'for care to be excellent staff need to be helpful, kind, caring, comforting, willing to spend time talking'.
3. Respect – 'listen to us, take an interest in us, do not ignore us, don't patronise us, consider our privacy'.
4. Some degree of choice about our care – 'this allows us to feel more in control, makes us feel valued'.
5. Explanations about what is happening to us – 'remember to tell us and not just our parents'.

If these indicators were found to reflect the views of children and young people in other countries, they could form the basis for international, client-centred standards of practice and for educational pathways for nurses and other health professionals caring for children.

The nursing profession

Commonalities

Common influences that shape nursing across the globe include the fact that most nurses are women and, therefore, the value given to nurses' work aligns with the position of women in society. In many countries, nursing is still a low status job with low wages and poor working conditions (WHO 1997). Elsewhere, nurses may be valued and supported by society but not paid at the same level as occupations with similar educational requirements. According to Evers (2004), nursing has one common and pivotal role no matter what the health care system is

> to guarantee organisational permanency in meeting the basic human needs of the patients (p. 23).

He states that 'compassion, respect and solidarity with the weak and persons in need were and still are the basic values of our profession'. These fundamental values and the shared focus of nursing practice on basic human needs are acknowledged in all definitions of nursing. Children's nursing has traditionally focused on helping the sick or injured child and the family to prevent and manage the physical, psychological, social, emotional and spiritual effects of the illness or injury and its treatment.

Nurses also supported investigation, diagnosis and treatment of disease by monitoring the effects of treatment, providing support to the child and family and promoting independence and self-care. These roles remain the core of children's nursing: working with the family to ensure the child's human needs are met as well as supporting, teaching and helping the child and family to manage the health problem.

Differences

A detailed analysis of nursing practice around the world was published by the WHO in 1997. Although the details may have changed in subsequent years, the factors that influence nursing practice remain the same. Evidence from the six geographic regions of the world illustrates the diverse scope of practice and nursing's flexibility in adapting to changes in need, new diseases, new technologies and evolving health care systems, balancing increasing specialisation with shifts to primary care and generalism. Health care reform is seen by nurse leaders in many countries both as an enabling and a constraining factor for the development of nursing roles and the quality of nursing practice (WHO 1997).

Nursing registration/regulatory authorities that exist in different forms in many countries are responsible for deciding the scope of nursing practice and appropriate educational preparation. However, the WHO report suggests that:

> the lack of power for nurses in policy making, the effect of gender and the transference of tasks from medicine to nursing may be far more influential (WHO 1997, p. 3).

The ICN advises national nursing associations to seek support in legislation that recognises the distinctive and autonomous nature of nursing practice (ICN 2004), but this assumes a level of leadership and influence that may not be present, even if such associations exist. There are differences in legal regulation, for example, in Germany, nurses are not obliged to register but the title 'nurse' is protected by law (Evers 2004). Other countries such as France, Italy and the Nordic countries have specific regulations covering responsibilities and competencies (WHO 1997). In Switzerland, the government has recognised the high cost of nursing services and its relative invisibility in national health statistics; data about nursing practice are now required at the national level by law (Institute for Health and Economics 2006).

Paediatric nursing in the Netherlands is largely 'regulated' by the Association of Paediatric Nurses, which has leadership positions on committees setting quality standards for practice and agreeing education curricula (Vereniging van kinderverpleegkundigen 2006). However, in most other countries where paediatric nursing associations exist, the position is very different as they have little or no power to influence even within the nursing profession, let alone to affect national or international policy.

In almost all countries, nurses are the largest group of health care workers, but what they do varies widely depending not just on the economic and environmental context but also on workforce factors such as nurse–doctor ratio and nursing numbers. In Europe, Finland and Sweden have the highest number of nurses with around 13 nurses per inhabitant (Evers 2004). The UK, Belgium, Denmark, Germany and the Netherlands have 8–9, and Greece has the lowest with just over 1 registered nurse per 1000 population (Evers 2004). In the US, Canada and other countries, researchers have demonstrated the critical importance of nurse staffing and skill mix to quality of care and patient safety in hospitals (Tourangeau *et al.* 2006).

Educational preparation differs between countries in every aspect from age at entry and the entry qualifications required to the level of qualification and the competencies achieved. The focus of nursing education also differs with some countries offering preparation as a general nurse and subsequent specialisation, for example, in midwifery, gerontology, children's or mental health nursing; a few countries offer these as direct entry or branch type programmes that follow a general introductory period. The Paediatric Nursing Associations of Europe (PNAE) specifies that a course of study should prepare the paediatric nurse to be able to:

- Deliver rights-based, holistic, child- and family-centred care.
- Promote physical and mental health and well-being.
- Provide nursing care of infant, child and adolescent with acute/chronic/ life-threatening/limiting physical and mental conditions, disability/impairment (physical/intellectual/sensory).

in all health care settings.

Courses preparing paediatric nurses must also include child protection and accident and disease prevention (PNAE 2004). In those countries that do have a children's or paediatric nursing qualification, this is most often offered after initial qualification and mostly self-funded. The UK, Belgium, Germany and, since 2001, Italy are among the few countries that offer a first level qualification in children's nursing. Until 1997, the general nurse in Italy cared for patients of all ages, and although there was a 1-year post-qualifying course for certification in children's nursing, the majority of nurses working in paediatrics did not hold this additional certificate. In 1997, a government decree defined the profile of children's nurse, and in 2001, specific education for children's nursing (3 years at university level) was started (PNAE 2006).

In contrast, Australian nurses argue against returning to a direct entry course, recommending that the child health content of basic nursing education be improved and barriers to specialty post-basic education removed:

> The number of nurses choosing to undertake such education is falling due to the barriers of cost, lack of recognition and competing demands on nurses' time. Consequently, there is a shortage of educated, experienced nurses in children's health care and the quality of health services for children and their families is in jeopardy (Australian Confederation of Paediatric and Child Health Nurses 2001, http://www.dest.gov.au/archive/highered/nursing/cub/62.rtf).

They also noted the threat to the educational preparation of future nurses and nurse specialists with fewer experienced clinical nurses to teach and support both undergraduate and postgraduate students.

To become a 'certified paediatric nurse' (CPN) in the US, a qualified nurse typically applies to work at a site with children's services, most of which offer classroom and clinical experience towards the CPN certification exam (Society of Pediatric Nurses 2006). A master's degree in nursing is required to become a paediatric nurse practitioner (PNP) or clinical nurse specialist in paediatrics. The nurse must apply to the relevant state board of nursing for recognition as an advanced practice nurse and take their respective exam for certification. In Canada, registered nurses can undertake post-qualifying paediatric courses such as the Advanced Specialty Certificate or Bachelor of Science in Pediatric Nursing depending on the requirements of the regulatory body of the province.

As in most other countries, community child health care is undertaken by generalist community nurses who have no additional education, and hospitals employ generalist nurses in child settings. Given this context where children's nursing is seen as a specialty, it is not surprising that there is very little further specialist education available to children's nurses; the UK is almost unique in the range of specific courses, for example, in children's cancer nursing or paediatric intensive care.

The extent to which nurses have authority and autonomy in decision making and practice is one of the most significant differences between countries. According to the WHO (1997) report, as nursing education is strengthened nurses should be more able to take independent care decisions. However, this also requires a change in attitudes towards nurses by doctors and managers, that is, seeing them as professional colleagues rather than as technical or skilled workers. It also requires changes in 'nurses' self image and increased in confidence in their own abilities' (WHO 1997, p. 101).

'*Degree of nursing practice autonomy*' is one of the factors addressed in a seminal analysis of nursing role development by Ketefian *et al.* (2001), which compares the development of advanced practice in four countries – Brazil, Thailand, the UK and the US. Critical elements for the evolution of advanced roles included inter/intra-professional collaboration, support of nursing leadership, educational infrastructure, support of government through policy and financing, and documentation on the effectiveness of the role. As a result of the numerous and complex factors that shape practice, nurses' roles differ widely across the globe. The dimensions that describe these differences are further explored in the discussion of children's nursing roles in the next section.

Children's nursing roles descriptions

General nursing role descriptions are presented in the literature using a number of different models, from lists of practice activities to competency frameworks. There are only few examples of role descriptions of children's nurses but a growing number about the role of PNPs, usually as part of studies evaluating their effectiveness.

The US National Association of Pediatric Nurse Practitioners (PNPs) implies two different roles depending on whether the nurse practitioner is working in primary care or as an acute care/specialty PNP.

Primary care PNPs:

- Provide health maintenance care for children, including well-child examinations.
- Perform routine developmental screenings.
- Diagnose and treat common childhood illnesses.
- Provide anticipatory guidance regarding common child health concerns.
- Provide childhood immunisations.
- Perform school physicals.

Acute care and speciality PNPs:

- Provide care to children who are acutely, chronically and critically ill.
- Perform in-depth physical assessments.
- Interpret results of laboratory and diagnostic tests.
- Order medications and perform therapeutic treatments in a variety of settings (National Association of Pediatric Nurse Practitioners 2006).

The Australian Confederation of Paediatric and Child Health Nurses (ACPCHN) makes a clear distinction between paediatric nurses and child health nurses. However, role descriptors in the form of competency standards apply to both with 'the emphasis of the role will be influenced by the context in which the nurse practices' (ACPCH 2004). This approach is also taken by the UK Nursing and Midwifery Council (NMC): the standards of proficiency for registration as a nurse are generic with those on branch programmes expected to achieve the same standards 'within the context of the area of practice' (NMC 2004).

In some Canadian provinces, as in many European countries, child health is separated from child illness and well-child services are provided by generalist primary care or community nurses (Canadian Nurses' Association 2005). Competencies for nurse practitioners in Ontario, for example, distinguish the role of the primary health care (family/all ages) nurse practitioner and the acute care (child) nurse practitioner who is 'usually in, but not limited to, hospital acute care inpatient or outpatient settings' (College of Nurses of Ontario 2006). Comprehensive descriptions of the children's nursing roles at different levels of expertise and in different specialties have been published by the Royal College of Nursing in the UK in the form of competency and role frameworks (RCN 2004).

From the detail of these examples, a number of dimensions emerge that can help identify differences in the roles of nurses caring for children in the same country as well as between countries. The dimensions are similar to the role development guidance introduced by the Royal College of Nursing paediatric oncology nurses' forum (Casey *et al.* 2001) and it includes the following:

1. Focus of care: child, family and whole community.
2. Domain of practice: health/illness (emphasis on one or both).
3. Scope of practice: medicine/nursing (emphasis on cure or care or both).
4. Location: hospital, community or crossing boundaries.
5. Specialty:
   - client group, for example, adolescents, neonates and children with disabilities.
   - clinical specialty such as diabetes, continence and mental health.
   - intervention type such as pain management.

Nursing roles can be described using these dimensions, but all roles will include many of these elements. For example, a nurse caring for children in a remote location will be required to address all aspects of child health and illness management in community, home and school. An expert children's diabetes nurse may include all locations, many interventions, every aspect of health promotion, medical investigation, drug prescribing and nursing care provided there is support from the multi-disciplinary team and sufficient numbers of skilled nurses to support this workload.

Conclusion

Comparing nursing roles is an important activity that can lead to a deeper understanding of how those roles are shaped and what could be done to change existing roles if these are not effective. However, merely describing differences does not tell us whether one approach is more effective than another. With very few exceptions, there are no evaluation data to support assumptions about how changed roles might support improvements in quality and cost-effectiveness in any field of nursing. An example from elderly care nursing shows just how important such data can be (Jensdottir *et al.* 2003). When quality indicators recorded in care homes in Iceland, Canada and the US were compared, significant differences were found in rates of incontinence, catheter use, tube feeding use, development of pressure ulcers, physical restraint use, residents with depression, residents spending little or no time in activities and falls. This mix of interventions and outcome indicators highlighted different clinical practices, which could account for differences in outcomes.

In 1974, WHO Europe set up a study that involved 23 centres in 11 European countries and investigated people's needs for nursing care (Ashworth *et al.* 1987). Its goal was to describe nursing practice so that it could be better planned and organised. Paediatric nursing associations and nurses across the globe need to group together to improve understanding about children's need for nursing care with good, comparative data about what makes that care effective. Working with and learning from children's nurses in other countries and from our nursing colleagues in other fields will help improve the quality of care for children, young people and families.

References

Ashworth P *et al.* (1987). *Nursing Care Summary of a European Study. A Study of People's Needs for Nursing Care and of the Planning, Implementation and Evaluation of Care Provided by Nurses in Two Selected Groups of People in the European Region.* Geneva: World health Organisation (WHO).

Australian Confederation of Paediatric and Child Health Nurses (ACPCH) (2001). *Submission to the National Review of Nursing Education.* http://www.dest.gov.au/archive/highered/nursing/sub/62.rtf (accessed 27 November 2006).

Australian Confederation of Paediatric and Child Health Nurses (ACPCH) (2004). *Minimum standards for nurses caring for children and young people.* http://www.acpchn.org.au/ (accessed 27 November 2006).

Bryce J, Boschi-Pinto C, Shibuya K, Black RE, WHO Child Health Epidemiology Reference Group (2005). WHO estimates of the causes of death in children. *Lancet*, 365, 1147–1152.

Canadian Nurses' Association (2005). *Children's health and nursing: A summary of the issues.* www.cna-nurses.ca/CNA/documents/pdf/publications/BG2_Childrens_Health_and_Nursing_e.pdf (accessed 27 November 2006).

Casey A, Gibson F and Hooker L (2001). Role development in children's nursing: Dimensions, terminology and practice framework. *Paediatric Nursing*, 13(2), 36–40.

College of Nurses of Ontario (2006). *Registered nurses in the extended class: Description of three streams of nurse practitioner practice.* www.cno.org/for/rnec/3streams.htm (accessed 27 November 2006).

Department for Education and Skills and Department of Health (2004). *Asthma Exemplar National Service Framework for Children, Young People and Maternity.* London: Department of Health.

Department for Education and Skills and Department of Health (2006). *Improving the Transition of Young People with Long Term Conditions from Children's to Adult Health Services.* London: Department of Health.

Department of Health (2003). *Getting the Right Start: National Service Framework for Children, Young People and Maternity Services: Standard for Hospital Services.* London: Department of Health.

Edwards P, Roberts I, Green J, Lutchmun S. (2006). Deaths from injury in children and employment status in family: analysis of trends of class specific death rates. *BMJ* 333, 119 (15 July) (Chap 4).

Evers G (2004). *The nurses' role present and future.* In: Tadd W (ed.), *Ethical and Professional Issues in Nursing: Perspectives from Europe.* Basingstoke: Palgrave.

Every Child Matters (2006). *Child and adolescent mental health services.* www.everychild-matters.gov.uk/health/camhs/ (accessed 27 November 2006).

Gillies A (2003). *What Makes a Good Healthcare System?* Oxford: Radcliffe.

Health Select Committee (1997). *Hospital services for children and young people. House of Commons Health Select Committee* (Session 1996–97) *Fifth Report.* HMSO, London.

Howe L, Huttly S and Abramsky T (2006). Risk factors for injuries in young children in four developing countries: The Young Lives Study. *Tropical Medicine and International Health,* 11(10), 1557–1566.

Institute for Health and Economics (2006). *Nursing data: The Swiss nursing project for the development of a Nursing Data System.* http://www.isesuisse.ch/nursingdata/ (accessed 10 November 2006).

International Council of Nurses (ICN) (2002). *Career Moves and Migration: Critical Questions.* Geneva: ICN.

International Council of Nurses (ICN) (2004). *Position Statement: Scope of Nursing Practice.* Geneva: ICN, www.icn.ch/psscope.htm.

International Council of Nurses (ICN) (2006). *Position Statement: Credentialing.* http://www.icn.ch/matters_credentialing.htm (accessed 10 November 2006).

Jensdottir AB, Rantz M and Hjaltadottir I *et al.* (2003). International comparison of quality indicators in United States, Icelandic and Canadian nursing facilities. *International Nursing Review,* 50(2), 79–84.

Ketefian S, Redman RW, Hanucharurnkul S, Masterson A and Neves EP (2001). The development of advanced practice roles: Implications in the international nursing community. *International Nursing Review,* 48, 152–163.

Lindeke L, Nakai M and Johnson L (2006). Capturing children's voices for quality improvement. *MCN American Journal of Maternal and Child Nursing,* 31(5), 290–295.

Moules T (2004). Whose quality is it? *Paediatric Nursing,* 16(6), 30–31.

National Association of Pediatric Nurse Practitioners (2006). *What do PNPs do?* http://www.napnap.org/index.cfm?page=15 (accessed 12 December 2006).

Nursing and Midwifery Council (NMC) (2004). *Standards of proficiency for pre-registration nursing education.* http://www.nmc-uk.org/aSection.aspx?SectionID=32 (accessed 12 December 2006).

Paediatric Nursing Associations of Europe (PNAE) (2005). *Definition of a paediatric nurse.* www2.rcn.org.uk/cyp/forums (accessed 27 November 2006).

Paediatric Nursing Associations of Europe (PNAE) (2006). *PNAE membership: Italy.* www2.rcn.org.uk/cyp/forums (accessed 27 November 2006).

Royal College of Nursing (RCN) (2004). *Services for children and young people: Preparing nurses for future roles.* London: RCN.

Samad L, Tate AR, Dezateux C, Peckham C, Butler N and Bedford H (2006). Differences in risk factors for partial and no immunisation in the first year of life: Prospective cohort study. *British Medical Journal,* 332, 1312–1313.

Sarajarvi A, Haapamaki ML and Paavilainen E (2006). Emotional and informational support for families during their child's illness. *International Nursing Review*, 53(3), 205–210.

Shields L and Nixon J (2004). Hospital care of children in four countries. *Journal of Advanced Nursing*, 45(5), 475–486.

Society of Pediatric Nurses (2006). *Becoming a pediatric nurse*. www.pedsnurses.org (accessed 27 November 2006).

Starfield B and Shi L (2002). Policy relevant determinants of health: An international perspective. *Health Policy*, 60(3), 201–218.

Stiller C, Desnades E, Danon S, Izarzuaza I, Ratiu A, Vasseleva-Valerianove Z and Steliariva-Foucher E (2006). Cancer incidence and survival in European adolescents (1978–1997). Report from the Automated Childhood Cancer Information System project. *European Journal of Cancer*, 42(13), 2006–2018.

Tourangeau AE, Cranley LA and Jeffs L (2006). Impact of nursing on hospital patient mortality: A focused review and related policy implications. *Quality and Safety in Health Care*, 15(1), 4–8.

UNICEF (2005). *The State of the World's Children 2006: Excluded and Invisible*. New York: UNICEF.

United Nations (UN) (1989). *Convention on the Rights of the Child*. Geneva: United Nations.

US Department of Health and Human Services (2006). *Child and adolescent mental health*. http://mentalhealth.samhsa.gov/child/ChildHealth.asp (accessed 27 November 2006).

Vereniging van kinderverpleegkundigen (2006). *The Dutch Association of Paediatric Nurses*. http://www.vvkv.nl/page.php?id=233 (accessed 27 November 2006).

Victorian Government (2006). *CAMHS in communities*. http://www.health.vic.gov.au/mentalhealth/publications/camhsrep0906.pdf (accessed 27 November 2006).

Werry Centre for Child and Adolescent Mental Health (2006). *About CAMHS*. http://www.werrycentre.org.nz (accessed 27 November 2006).

WHO Europe (2005). *The European Health Report 2005: Public Health Action for Healthier Children and Populations*. WHO regional office for Europe, Copenhagen.

WHO Nursing/Midwifery Health Systems Development Programme (1997). *Nursing Practice Around the World*. Geneva: WHO.

Wilimas JA, Donahue N, Chammas G, Fouladi M, Bowers LJ and Ribeiro RC (2003). Training subspecialty nurses in developing countries: Methods, outcome, and cost. *Medical and Pediatric Oncology*, 41(2), 136–140.

Part 2
The Registered Practitioner in Nursing: Scope of Practice

Introduction

Jane Hughes

Part 2 examines many aspects of practice for registered practitioners in nursing, ranging from acute care settings to children's nurses developing roles in primary care, public health, mental health and children and young people (CYP) with disabilities. These chapters include valuable insights from practising children's nurses in the form of case studies; the contributions include newly and recently qualified children's nurses from acute care and community settings, experienced practitioners from children's community nursing and the field of disability nursing. The chapters on public health and mental health demonstrate examples of working with CYP in a range of settings, which would help the reader to consider the wider application of public health and supporting the mental health of CYP.

The final chapter in this section written by a specialist nurse in child protection aims to address some of the key current issues in this field. It includes some scenarios that reflect some of the significant dilemmas that nurses caring for CYP may encounter with regard to safeguarding CYP. There is a strong focus on multidisciplinary working and the need for clear communication channels between the various agencies that come into contact with CYP and their families.

Chapter 4

The Newly Qualified Registered Practitioner in Acute Settings

Sarah Moxon and Geraldine Lyte

Introduction

Given the importance which is now placed on child health in our society, Jeremy Jolley's historical analysis in Chapter 1 shows us that acute children's nursing, or nursing children and young people (CYP) in a hospital setting, has a surprisingly short history. Indeed, it was not until the damaging effect of industrialisation that public attention was roused to the appalling health of children in UK (Brookes and Hawarth 1993, Webster 2001). It was consequently only towards the middle of the 19th century that the notion of child health or paediatrics as a separate entity was really introduced (Platt 1959). Before this, childhood illness was regarded as highly contagious, incurable and dangerous (Barnes 1999, Pelling 1998). The gradual transition towards improved child health services, as shown in Chapter 2, has concurred with a role for nurses trained specifically to look after the needs of sick children.

Over the past few decades, the role of the children's nurse has seen significant developments, and it is both an interesting and fast moving time for all those involved in child health. The tremendous decrease in childhood mortality in the past half-century has simultaneously seen an increase in childhood morbidity, particularly in chronic disease management (Hendrick *et al.* 1998), as well as current day issues such as increased childhood obesity (Chinn and Rona 2001, Chinn *et al.* 2005), allergic diseases (Burney and Jarvis 1998) and teenage pregnancy (Kane and Wellings 1999). There is thus an even greater need for trained professionals to treat and care for CYP and their families through periods of ill health. The focus of children's nursing on ill health has changed however. The titles 'Children's Nurse', 'Paediatric Nurse' or 'Children's and Young People's Nurse' have replaced what was originally referred to on the nursing register as the 'Sick Children's Nurse'. The latter title assumed a child must be sick to be nursed, whereas the 21st century children's nurse is recognised as having involvement in every aspect of a CYP's growth and development.

In this chapter, we will draw on the work presented in the first three chapters of this book to examine what challenges newly qualified registered children's nurses currently face. Our focus will be on the acute care setting and the early experiences of the first author (Sarah Moxon) following her graduation as a children's nurse. In Chapter 5, Lucy Andrews and Amber Barnum examines such challenges faced by newly qualified children's nurses in primary care. To avoid confusion, throughout this chapter we will use the term 'children's nurse' as the term to refer to any nurse prepared specifically to care for babies and CYP.

Acute care children's nursing

It has been highlighted in Chapters 1 and 2 that Dr Charles West is generally considered as one of the earliest influential character in paediatrics, particularly with regard to children's nursing. He recognised there was a real difference needed in the approach to caring for children in place of adults and was one of the founders of the first children's hospital in the UK at Great Ormond Street in 1852. His 1908 text on '*How to Nurse Sick Children*' read:

> I would not advise anyone whose temper is fretful, or whose spirits are low, to undertake the office of a [children's] nurse (p. 3).

As early as 1900, the principal role of the children's nurse was considered to be recognising signs of illness and caring for and observing sick children. Nurses were required to be:

> able to read and write with facility and should attend to the children with care and kindness and use every endeavour to make them happy. Should a nurse fail in these respects, or show impatience or ill-temper, she shall render herself liable for dismissal... (Hospital Constitution Queen Elizabeth Hospital for Children, 1874, p. 3).

It was in this era that emphasis on the quality of nursing care first included the association of quality nursing on difference in outcomes for these acutely sick children (West 1854). Since that time, medical and scientific advances, especially in the establishment of antibiotics and immunisation programmes, have seen a massive reduction in childhood mortality from what used to be regarded as fatal infectious diseases (Rivett 1998).

More recent changes in local populations and lifestyles associated with factors such as nutrition, immigration, reduced infant and childhood mortality and CYP mental health have given rise to a plethora of disorders that bring CYP into the acute care setting. A number of these disorders have not been formerly associated as a major concern with CYP (such as obesity and type II diabetes) or are relatively new to the UK (such as thalassaemia and sickle cell disease); (Thomas-Hope 1992). Furthermore, a host of inherited disorders and malignancies can be diagnosed and treated more successfully in acute care settings in the first instance, including leukaemia and cystic fibrosis (DH 2004). Disability, neurological disorders and recognition of illness or injury resulting from physical, emotional or sexual abuses of CYP are also better understood and treated. This is reflected today with the growing concern regarding CYP abuse and the need for more rigorous child assessment, protection and expanding paediatric children's and adolescent mental health services (CAMHS) (DFES 2003, DH 2004).

Four key documents have been published in the past 6 years, which have had a considerable impact on the way in which we nurse CYP:

- Learning from Bristol/Kennedy Report (DH 2001).
- *Victoria Climbie Inquiry* (Laming 2003).
- The National Service Framework for Children and Young People (NSF) (DH 2004).
- Every Child Matters (DFES 2003).

Conclusions drawn from these publications stipulate over and again that acute children's nursing needs to be CYP centred and highly integrated with other CYP services. Nurses need to listen to and work in negotiation and partnership with CYP and their families and carers, and early intervention is crucial. A greater focus on early health promotion, teaching and management for acutely ill CYP, initiated in acute care settings, is intended to steer children's services as much as possible into community and primary care settings and also into prevention of further physical, social and emotional pathology (DH 2004).

So the health of children today is now more subject to ongoing investigation and audit, and this has been facilitated greatly since 2004 by the publication of the NSF (DH 2004). It is against this backdrop of advances and change that acute care children's services are currently premised on a rapid turnaround of assessment, diagnosis and initial treatment for CYP, to place the main focus of their longer term health care, whatever their needs, at home with their families and carers (DH 2004, Health care Commission 2007).

Children's nurses in acute care are increasingly regarded as frontline staff, and therefore, newly qualified nurses need to adapt to this new, more dynamic, role through a commitment to lifelong learning and self-development, application of evidence-based research and inter-professional and multidisciplinary collaboration. Because of this, newly qualified children's nurses who join acute care services, like their general nurse counterparts, need to be prepared to deal with a greater throughput of acutely ill CYP with often complex health needs, which require more sophisticated clinical reasoning and decision-making skills than ever before (Jackson 2005, Mohammed and Trigg 2006).

The transition from student to nurse

In 1999, the Department of Health (DH) and later the United Kingdom Central Council for Nursing, Midwifery and Health Visiting (UKCC) – which became the Nursing and Midwifery Council (NMC) in 2002 – published new education and workplace proposals for nurses (DH 1999, UKCC 1999). The recommendations from these publications were incorporated into National Health Service (NHS) reforms emanating from the government's *Modernisation* agenda, most notably in the NHS Plan (DH 2000).

The NHS Plan (DH 2000) represents a 10-year strategy to reform health care and place care *around the patient* (p. 10). It recommended that nurses undertake a wider range of clinical responsibilities, supported by the new DH model of education and training, titled *Making a Difference* (DH 1999). The impact of this on nursing was to shift attention from delineating boundaries for nursing practice to a guiding principle of multi-skilled health professionals, including nurses, who could meet the requirements of health service users at increasingly advanced levels of practice (DH 2000). The net effect for nursing education has been to focus attention on how well pre-registration programmes can prepare students for immediate working life, lifelong learning and career development, following guidelines for higher education levels from the DH (1999) education model and the UKCC Commission for Education's recommendations (UKCC 1999).

In 2005, Sarah Moxon, co-author of this chapter, graduated as a registered children's nurse with a Bachelor of Nursing (Hons) (BN) degree from the University of Manchester. Her cohort, which commenced in 2002, was the first to experience a revised curriculum following recommendations from the DH (1999) and the UKCC (1999). It had also been redesigned to facilitate development of students' potential for innovation and leadership more explicitly and to map the programme against the QAA Benchmark Statement for undergraduate nursing programmes (QAAHE 2001).

In the summer of 2005, there was much anticipation of the programme's impending conclusion among Sarah and her peers, their mentors and lecturers. This anticipation was captured as part of a 4-year qualitative case study by Geraldine Lyte, co-author of this chapter, into undergraduate nursing students' development and employability (Lyte 2007). The study had involved adult and child branch students from Sarah's cohort, mentors, lecturers, practice educators, lead nurses from local trusts and personnel involved in strategic planning and purchasing for nursing education.

In the study, students, mentors and lecturers in particular referred to factors interrelated with increasing workplace responsibilities such as students' confidence to practice as a registered nurse, especially in terms of mastery and application of technical skills and in independent clinical reasoning and judgement. Other expectations of newly qualified nurses in the study included independent management of care generally, positive self-efficacy and lifelong learning and development potential.

Early employment issues that emerged from Sarah's cohort included preceptorship, post-qualifying skills development, finding employment in an area one could feel comfortable in as a staff nurse and wider employment choices. The students from the 2002 BN cohort registered in the autumn of

2005, just a few months prior to changes in the NHS that saw a change of employment opportunities for newly qualified nurses (BBC News 2007). By the time they were halfway through their final placement (May/June 2005), most students who had applied for posts after they qualified had been successful.

Employment choices ranged from full-time employment in acute care settings in Great Britain and Canada (*n*=1 *student who was a Canadian national*), community nursing, agency nursing, working abroad and taking time out. Several of the new graduates gained rotational posts whereby they moved to three or four different units within a trust in their first post-qualifying year. They regarded these posts as giving them an advantage for extending their skills portfolio and professional self-efficacy beliefs, thus enhancing their future employability potential. A few of the graduates obtained posts in specialised settings, such as intensive care, some of whom had decided on their focus within the first year of their undergraduate programme.

Sarah's experiences as a newly qualified nurse will now be reflected in a short case study.

Being a newly qualified children's nurse in acute care

A year into my working career, I have been given the opportunity to contribute to this chapter. I have contributed to all aspects of its preparation, in particular by offering a discussion of my experiences as a newly qualified practitioner in the acute setting. Over that year, and subsequently, I have had the privilege of seeing CYP whom I have cared for overcome wide-ranging diseases and other pathology and at the same time grow and develop. Some of the very tiny babies that I watched through the windows of an incubator are now sitting, standing and smiling. My case study in this chapter aims to shed some light on the current role of the newly qualified children's nurse in acute care. It will include a reflection on some of my personal experiences, expectations and developments.

There has been massive upheaval and financial difficulties within the NHS in the past few years, and this has created a challenging climate to enter the profession. I have found, for example, that pressures on nurses and other health professionals from developments such as the changes in junior doctors' roles (McBride 2004) have sometimes tested the positive attitude that newly qualified nurses are expected to bring to the workplace. In writing this case study, I have attempted to bring together my experiences with an objective stance and tie together the reality of that experience with my own optimism for my career as a children's nurse. My aim has been to provide a perspective that may be useful to professionals at all levels of children's nursing.

I decided to move to London to commence a newly qualified rotational programme for children's nurses, which gave me the opportunity to work in a number of different trusts and settings. East London offers a backdrop of immense diversity, and so in terms of child health care, it provides the opportunity to witness and to help treat rare pathological conditions among a range of different social and ethnic groups and the resulting health problems from these conditions. In a number of works by Charles Dickens, he described the east end as a densely populated maze of mean and dirty streets. The contemporary population of Hackney, however, is young, expanding, highly mobile and culturally diverse. Almost half of Hackney's secondary pupils, for example, speak English as a second language. Health conditions that might be assumed as rare in other demographic areas in the UK, such as sickle cell disease, are more commonplace. I also feel that despite the challenges presented by working in such a busy, built-up inner city area, it propels practitioners in acute care health settings to be creative and resourceful in the care that they offer. In my own experience, it is simultaneously frustrating and sometimes overwhelming.

On the one hand, this experience has helped to form the practitioner I am today, though it has also had a detrimental effect on my confidence at times. However, there are other demands that impact on the professional nursing role, which have conflicted with my early aspirations as a children's nurse. This conflicting experience is that which is associated with increasing administration that moves registered practitioners further away from the traditional 'hands-on-care' that West and his contemporaries considered so vital to the traditional children's nurses role (Mohammed and Trigg 2006).

Many nurses, including myself, are sometimes concerned that the traditional nursing role has become blurred, with technicians, students and health care assistants having increasingly delegated nursing duties form parts of their roles. However, I have had the distinction of working with professional role models. They have helped me to combine a balance between developing and retaining the basic skills of acute care children's nursing practice, with organisational, academic and evidence-based learning and skills development, the combination which, I hope, will enable me to contribute to, and make a difference in, future child health nursing practice.

So, on what I consider to be a 'typical' general paediatric ward, such as where I held on my first post in an acute setting, the scope of problems CYP present with includes the following:

- The need for treatment of chronic conditions.
- The need for routine and emergency surgery.
- The need for care pre- or post-high dependency or intensive care.
- Management of acute onset of illness (such as gastroenteritis and respiratory illness).
- Caring for CYP with long-term health needs or special needs.
- Caring for CYP with cancer.
- CYP in need of outpatient services.
- Caring for CYP with intravenous (IV) therapy and pain relief.
- Orthopaedics.

- Palliative care and care of the dying CYP.
- Caring for CYP with mental health problems.
- Caring for CYP with varying social problems.

The health needs listed above can also include important referrals to other appropriate services (e.g. physiotherapy, speech and language, social or legal services or education).

Nursing skills are varied and dependent on experience, education and training, locality and trust policy. For example, some trusts are working to give greater autonomy and skill base to nurses through the creation of more specialised positions (e.g. Child Protection Nurse and Tissue Viability nurses). The skill mix is vital to the smooth running of acute care wards on a day-to-day basis, and from my initial experiences, I have found that a basic team normally consists of the following:

- Modern matron or ward manager.
- Senior sisters.
- Sisters.
- Senior staff nurses.
- Staff nurses (including newly qualified practitioners).
- Play therapists.
- Nursery nurses.
- Health care assistants and other support staff.
- Student nurses.

The support offered by the acute general CYP ward is founded in family-centred care, which in turn is based on negotiation and partnership with CYP and their families. Many CYP wards across the country base their philosophy for nursing on Anne Casey's partnership and negotiation model (Casey 1988), which has been an inspiration in the past 20 years for recovering the ideology of child/family-centred care proposed by Charles West and Catherine Wood (see Chapter 1, Jolley).

Underpinned by this philosophy, acute care children's nurses' skills will include CYP assessment, nursing diagnosis, planning, implementing and evaluating care, most importantly making clinical judgements and decisions with or on behalf of our CYP clients. Within this, some of the common intervention skills that are applied, from my experience, include the administration of medicines and controlled drugs, pre- and post-surgical care, pain relief, feeding [IV, bolus, oral, nasogastric (NG), bottle feeds and supporting breastfeeding], administration of nebulisers and oxygen therapy. Other skills include a complex combination of health promotion, parent/carer education, support and counselling, ensuring appropriate referrals, observing patients' physical and other status, accurate recording of observations and taking appropriate action. Here is an extract from my reflective working diary, which I wrote when I had been in practice for a few months. It exemplifies aspects of my development and dilemmas as a newly qualified practitioner.

Extract from a reflective working diary

In the past 6 months I have learnt to adapt as a registered nurse, from being a 'skilled professional' to a grafter!! First, I can be inserting a nasogastric tube, then cleaning the floor or unblocking the macerator in the sluice. Sometimes I feel like a secretary, then sometimes a counsellor. I can spend one day making endless phone calls to social workers, and another day unpacking pharmacy boxes and then another day caring for a high dependency child and their parents, leaving the room only to set up infusion pumps, and draw up IV antibiotics.

In my day at work, I rarely get the chance to say 'that, is not my job' because if the situation is there it must be dealt with. I have learnt how to put a leg in skin traction whilst singing along to the 'tweenies', 'wrestle' with drunken teenagers on Saturday nights, calm angry parents, deal with facetious surgeons, unprofessional hospital staff and crying mothers (sometimes simultaneously). I have looked after children with *run-of-the-mill* viruses and then rare complex metabolic disorders, syndromes and disabilities; some children that are not physically sick; and some children that are very ill. I have learnt that without extensive resources, it is necessary to add some creativity to the care you offer and approach situations with openness and some sort of sense of humour.

As emphasised by the NSF (DH 2004), the role of the children's nurse is set to become more dynamic. The focus is not on ill health alone but also on preventative action and holistic care; children's nurses are becoming more involved in every aspect of a CYP and family's growth and development. This is dependent on having an adequately resourced educated and motivated workforce. Consequently, it places a great deal of pressure on the individual nurse, new to their fully accountable role. Finding your role as a children's nurse, thus, is a process, rather than an event, and in practice, this process can be at the same time exhilarating, confusing and intangible, particularly when faced with varying levels of support (Jackson 2005). This is exemplified in a further extract from my diary.

Further extract from a reflective working diary

The first 3 months were undoubtedly the hardest. Initially, it is a very steep learning curve; sometimes, I was well supported and at other times I felt totally unsupported. It is sometimes easy to forget how a single situation can revert into a total personal crisis where you question who you are, what you are doing and whether you can even begin to cope with the task in hand.

The critical thinking role of the children's nurse

As we noted earlier, nursing involves critical thinking through assessment, clinical reasoning, clinical judgements and clinical decision making. This is achieved in nursing practice through nursing process. Hockenberry and Wilson (2007) outline the nursing process as involving a series of interrelated, non-linear steps, typically referred to as assessment, diagnosis, planning, implementation and evaluation. Sarah has amended these slightly to fit into how she has developed her own approach to providing care for CYP and their families and carers.

Assessment, diagnosis and planning

Collecting patient data, identifying the problems and needs of the CYP, establishing a nursing diagnosis, developing a care plan.

Implementation

With the CYP and family/carer, initiating and putting into action the interventions identified; attempting to base practice on evidence-based skills and individual CYP clients' specific needs.

Evaluation

Evaluate effectiveness of the applied intervention and progress of action. Question if action has achieved desired outcomes, if not what outcome has been achieved and why.

Documentation

Record what has been carried out in as much detail as possible, in collaboration with the CYP and family/carer.

Reflection

Reflect on the preceding events, actions and the outcomes; how the situation could be improved or changed; how it could be approached differently in the future – trying to avoid feelings of guilt and frustration and focus on positives. The very nature of nursing means the outcome will not always be favourable.

Here is an example of how Sarah applied her critical thinking skills through her nursing process with a particular child and family.

I was assigned an 18-month-old patient who had been admitted for observation and NG feeding due to dehydration and poor weight gain. On assessment, he was noticeably small for his age and underweight. His mother was understandably anxious. Planning involved treating his immediate medical needs (basic observations and give prescribed medications); I also planned to observe his feeding and encourage appropriate oral feeds. A referral to the speech and language team and the dietician was needed in that they could come and see the patient on the ward to support his mother. He would also need a community referral. Medically he was an undemanding patient as he had few medications and no immediate acute medical needs, as he was now well hydrated (after 2 days of NG feeding) and clinically stable.

On the ward round, it was decided that the NG tube should be removed and the patient discharged. I was concerned about the decision, as I did not feel that the patient's needs had been met and the mother was very distressed and worried about going home. I was unable to reach the speech and language team and bleeped the dietician who said she would see the patient in the afternoon. I removed the NG tube (somewhat reluctantly) and gave the child's mother a range of age-appropriate foods to give him.

Hours later he had not touched any of the food and had only drank very small amounts of milk. Senior members of staff were keen to discharge him imminently as his needs were not acute. This was a difficult situation, my own judgement, as the child's nurse was that he was not ready for discharge without an appropriate assessment from a dietician and speech and language therapist. Furthermore, I had not seen him eating and drinking and did not feel that this met appropriate criteria for discharge. Instead, I kept him in the bay and re-called the dietician and the speech and language therapist to explain the situation. They were immediately concerned and offered to come to see the patient as a priority. Both of them felt that there was need for further investigation; they felt there was a possibility of a problem of long-term reflux causing oral aversion and that the patient needed to continue NG feeds until an appropriate feeding plan was in place to slowly introduce oral feeds. This would mean another night in hospital to re-introduce the NG tube and teach the child's mother how to use the feeding pump so she could be discharged to care for him at home under the supervision of the community team.

Assessment, diagnosis and planning

The child needs adequate nutrition and his prescribed medicines; his mother also needs support. At the decision for discharge, discharge preparation and appropriate referrals need to be made. Conflict arises when the nursing diagnosis I have made and the assessment of the patient's needs differs from that dictated by a senior staff.

Implementation

Basing nursing care using my learned skills and evidence-based interventions. Offer a variety of age-appropriate foods, encourage food play and try to talk to the patient's mother about normal family habits and eating patterns. Contact multidisciplinary team (dietician and speech and language therapist).

Evaluation

A constant process. Is this intervention working? Am I offering appropriate care specific to this child and their family's needs? Is this child ready for discharge? Are they eating appropriately? Will the child be safe to be discharged home? Is effective communication occurring between the multidisciplinary team given that I have yet been unable to contact the speech and language team and the dietician and I am personally unsure of the decision for discharge? Should I have removed the NG tube?

At any point, the process can return to assessment and planning again.

Documentation

Sometimes the most frustrating and time consuming of all of the nursing process! Nevertheless, it is crucial to evidence how the plan of care is progressing, even though it often means staying late after the shift to finish all the paperwork. On a positive note, with practice, it becomes (slightly) quicker!

Reflection

Sometimes the skill is to learn how to learn from reflection. The above account provides a perfect example of some of the dilemmas faced by the newly qualified nurse when trying to make clinical judgments and decisions that will enhance a client's recovery. Underneath there is a desire to act autonomously and not from the direction of a senior staff, but in reality, there is often a need to balance growing autonomy with support and direction from those who have more experience and insight into CYP acute care.

On reflection, one of the easiest ways to minimise potential conflict and miscommunication is to ensure that the nurse caring for the CYP is always present in the room on the ward round, when the majority of the decisions for that day are made. Nurses often have vital insight into patient behaviour that is overlooked by other members of the Multidisciplinary team (MDT) who have less presence in the ward and thus the interactions and observations that take place. Perhaps this, aside from everything else, is one of the most important aspects of development of appropriate clinical judgment and decision-making skills as a staff nurse.

Summary

To summarise, this chapter has shown that demographic changes and their consequences in the health and welfare needs of CYP have had a profound effect on the role of contemporary children's nurses in acute care and, by consequence, on the expectations of newly qualified children's nurses. We have shown, for example, that factors such as preterm infants' survival rates have improved exponentially as intensive care technology has improved (Cooper *et al.* 1998). However, this in turn has increased demand for more highly skilled staff, neonatal intensive care facilities and, long-term follow-up and care resources to manage chronic illness sequelae resulting from prematurity and intensive care (Petrou 2003). Other demographic trends such as high numbers of teenage pregnancies in England (Tripp and Viner 2005), obesity among children (Ebbeling *et al.* 2002), the costs of more sophisticated technology and treatments, increased access to health care information and changing expectations add to this.

The ensuing widespread health care reform and modernisation has also placed greater demand on the need for more nurses with higher order intellectual skills that can be applied to clinical judgment and decision making, policy implementation, leadership and change management. Sarah's insightful account into her own beginnings as a registered children's nurse highlights just some of the dilemmas and challenges facing acute care children's nurses. On balance we hope that, ultimately, this chapter portrays what a positive, rewarding and challenging career exists within acute care children's nursing.

References

Barnes P (1999) Rural Manchester Children's Hospital 'Pendlebury' 1829–1999. Manchester: Churnet Valley Books.

BBC News (2007). *Nurse union condemns job cuts*. Available at: http://news.bbc.co.uk/1/hi/health/6552249.stm (25th September 2007).

Brookes A and Hawarth B (1993). *Boom Town Manchester 1800–1850*. Manchester: Portico Library.

Burney P and Jarvis D (1998). The epidemiology of allergic disease. *British Medical Journal*, 316(7131), 607–610.

Casey A (1988). A partnership with child and family, *Senior Nurse*, 8(4), 8–9.

Chinn S and Rona R (2001). Prevalence and trends in overweight and obesity in three cross sectional studies of British children 1974–1994, *British Medical Journal*, 322, 24–26.

Chinn S, Falascheti E, Primatesta P, Rona R and Stamatakis E (2005). Overweight and Obesity Trends from 1974–2003 in English Children: What is the role of socioeconomic factors? *Archives of Diseases in Childhood*, 90, 999–1004.

Cooper TR, Berseth CL, Adams JM and Weisman LE (1998). Actuarial survival in the premature infant less than 30 weeks' gestation *Pediatrics*, 101(6), 975–978.

Department for Education and Skills (DFES) (2003). *Every Child Matters*. London: HMSO.

Department of Health (DH) (1999). *Making a Difference: Strengthening the Nursing, Midwifery and Health Visiting Contribution to Health and Health Care*. London: HMSO.

Department of Health (DH) (2000). *The NHS Plan*. London: HMSO.

Department of Health (DH) (2001). *Learning From Bristol: The Report of the Public Inquiry into Children's Heart Surgery at Bristol Royal Infirmary from 198–1995*. London: HMSO.

Department of Health (DH) (2004). *National Service Framework for Children, Young People and Maternity Services*. www.dh.gov.uk/childrensnsf.

Ebbeling CB, Pawlak DB and Ludwig DS (2002). Childhood obesity: Public-health crisis, common sense cure. *The Lancet*, 360(9331), 473–482.

Health care Commission (2007). *Improving Services for Children in Hospital*. London: Commission for Health care and Audit Inspection.

Hendrick J, Moules T and Ramsey J (1998). *The Textbook of Children's Nursing*. Oxford: Nelson Homes.

Hockenberry M and Wilson D (2007). Wong's *Nursing Care of Infants and Children*, 8th edn. St Louis: Mosby-Elsevier.

Jackson K (2005).The roles and responsibilities of newly qualified children's nurses. *Paediatric Nursing*, 17(6), 26.

Kane R and Wellings K (1999). Trends in teenage pregnancy in England and Wales: How can we explain them? *Journal of the Royal Society of Medicine*, 92(6), 277–282.

Laming H (2003). *The Victoria Climbie Inquiry*. London: HMSO.

Lyte G (2007). *Graduateness in Nursing: A Case Study of Undergraduate Nursing Students' Development and Employability*. PhD Thesis (unpublished), The University of Manchester, The John Rylands University Library of Manchester.

McBride A (2004). *EU Directive Drives Reform of Junior Doctors' Working Hours*. http://www.eiro.eurofound.eu.int/about/2004/04/feature/uk0404105f.html (21st June 2004).

Mohammed T and Trigg E (2006). *Practices in Children's Nursing Guidelines for Hospital and Community*. Edinburgh: Churchill Livingstone.

Platt H (1959). *The Welfare of Children in Hospital*. London: Ministry of Health, Central Health Services Council.

Pelling M (1998). *The Common Lot: Sickness, Medical Occupation and the Urban Poor in Early Modern England*. London: Longman.

Petrou S (2003). Economic consequences of preterm birth and low birth-weight. *BJOG: An International Journal of Obstetrics and Gynaecology*, 110(20), 17–23.

(The) Quality Assurance Agency for Higher Education (QAAHE) (2001). *Benchmark Statement: Health Care Programmes*. Gloucester: QAAHE.

Rivett G (1998). *From Cradle to Grave: Fifty Years of the NHS*. London: Kings Fund.

Thomas-Hope EM (1992). International Migration and Health: Sickle Cell and Thalaesiamia health care in the UK. *Geojournal*, 26(1), 75–79.

Tripp J and Viner R (2005). Sexual health, contraception, and teenage pregnancy. *British Medical Journal*, 330(7491): 590–593.

United Kingdom Central Council for Nursing, Midwifery and Health Visiting (UKCC) (1999). *Fitness for Practice*. London: UKCC.

Webster C (2001). *Caring for Health: History and Diversity* (Health and Diseases Series Book 6). Buckingham: Open University Press.

West C (1854). *How to Nurse Sick Children* (reprinted). London: Longman.

West C (1908). *How to Nurse Sick Children*. London: Longmans, Green & co.

Chapter 5

The Newly Qualified Practitioner in Primary Care

Lucy Andrews and Amber Barnum

Introduction

Community Children's Nursing (CCN) services are now an established feature of children's health care. Their development has been underpinned by the commitment of experienced and highly skilled children's nurses, with a passion for caring for children in the community. A relatively new phenomenon within this has been to employ junior nurses within the CCN service. In this chapter, we will look at how one such service introduced a newly qualified nurse into a Community Children's Team. A reflective account of the experiences of one such nurse, Amber (co-author of this chapter), will be included. Changes in working practices, recommendations for practice, and opportunities for career progression will also be discussed.

The term 'child' alludes to any child or young person from birth to 18 years of age. A 'newly qualified nurse' in this context is any nurse who has been registered as a children's nurse for <12 months. All nurses are referred to in feminine terms; however, it is recognised that a proportion of nursing colleagues are male.

Development of CCN teams

Community services for children have been slow to develop despite historic recommendations from the Platt report that children should be nursed at home where possible (Ministry of Health 1959).

Since Sir Harry Platt's recommendations (Ministry of Health 1959), there has been increasing support for CCN; most notably, the formation of the CCN Forum within the Royal College of Nursing (RCN) in 1988 who became champions and a 'voice' for the expansion of CCN services. A National Health Service (NHS) executive took up the cause in 1996 with the document 'Child Health in the Community' (NHS Executive 1996), which strongly recommended the provision of skilled nursing care for children at home. The House of Commons

Health Committee (1997) advanced the profile of CCN and endorsed that all children, nationwide, should have access to such a service. Most recently, the National Service Framework for Children (2004) and Young People (NSF) offered for the first time an overarching national policy for children's services. This demonstrated a shift in political attitude to the rights and well-being of children (Mountford *et al.* 2005). The NSF sets out standards for the provision of health services for children and recommends that services be designed around the needs of the child, thus endorsing the ethos that sick children are best cared for at home wherever possible (Standard 6 p 33). Primary Care providers are responsible for ensuring that the NSF is implemented, which is encouraging for the development, planning and commissioning of CCN teams. It therefore makes strategic sense to nurture newly qualified children's nurses to become skilled and qualified in CCN.

In accordance with this, pilot schemes such as the Diana Teams (ENB and DH 1999) and more recently the New Opportunity Fund (2002) supported the role of the CCN in pioneering such services. From this, there has been a rapid development of CCN teams nationwide (RCN Forum). It is encouraging to note that in the most recent *Directory of Community Children's Nursing* (RCN 2004), 80% of children and families within the UK now have access to a CCN service. It is recognised, however, that there are stark variations in service provision from region to region (Eaton 2001). Teams may consist of anything from one part-time nurse to a comprehensive multidisciplinary team consisting of many team members, which may include professionals such as Occupational Therapists, Family Support Workers and Play Specialists.

Part of the reason for such variations is that CCN teams have typically been developed in response to local needs and will thus employ individual models of care and working practices (Eaton 2001, Drew *et al.* 2002). Caseloads can vary from children requiring only short-term interventions such as wound care and administration of medicines at home to children who require years of complex nursing care management. Quite often, it is the way in which a service has been developed which affects the type of services that are provided. Consequently, CCN practice has a wide remit in response to local service requirements and demographic factors. Nevertheless, Whiting (1998) has captured the core scope of care provided though CCN services, categorised as follows:

- Providing neonatal and post-neonatal care for infants requiring oxygen at home and long-term management of problems arising as a result of prematurity.
- Supporting children who have acute nursing needs including septic episodes and pneumonia. Facilitating early supported discharge is key in this category.
- Supporting children undergoing planned surgery such as scoliosis repair or hip reconstruction.
- Supporting children with long-term nursing needs such as cystic fibrosis, cancer, constipation (a proportion of these children will be 'technology dependent').

- Supporting and follow up children requiring emergency treatment such as burns, scalds and bites. Again, facilitating an early discharge or preventing admission is key here.
- Supporting children who have a disability and their families. CCNs will provide a service to children who have an ongoing nursing need. Again, a significant proportion of these children will be technology dependent.
- Supporting children with end of life/palliative care needs and their families.

CCN Teams may provide a combination of some or all of these services, which shapes the constitution of each team. Cramp *et al.* (2003) conducted a national survey to ascertain the characteristics of the provision of home nursing to children. Questionnaires were sent out to CCN teams nationally; 152 of 301 were returned completed. The results of this work indicated that teams who cared for children with chronic illness were staffed mainly by senior nurses (G grade/Band 6 nurses); however, these services tended to have nurses in specialist (senior) roles such as asthma or oncology. In contrast, teams that had a more acute focus to their care had a greater skill mix within the team, employing D and E grade/Band 5 nurses. This is pertinent when considering how the newly qualified nurse fits into the CCN team. Tatman and Jones (2005) advised that skill mix within CCN teams should be tailored to meet the needs of the children requiring the service.

Overview of the author's CCN team

The CCN team in question runs a multidisciplinary, generic, community-based service, which offers acute care support, and nurse-led clinics, complex, long-term health care management and palliative/end of life care. The team also incorporates a specialist service for children with chronic fatigue syndrome (CFS) and children who have continuing care needs. As stated previously, this is likely to be a unique service, responding to local need. The key to this service's expansion can be related to the procurement of government money to set up pilot schemes such as the Diana Team in 1999, providing care for children with life-threatening and life-limiting illness, and also initiatives to set up a service for children with CFS. These initiatives have a profound affect on the structure of the caseload. A significant proportion of these children will have complex health care needs and/or be 'technology dependent'.

Wagner (1988) offered the most widely recognised definition of technology dependence, stating that these are children 'who need both a medical device to compensate for the loss of a vital bodily function and substantial and ongoing nursing care to avert death or disability'.

There are many factors that have contributed to an increase in the ability to care for these children at home, including advances in medicine (especially neonatology) and invention of sophisticated portable medical equipment (such as ventilators), making discharge home and integration into the usual systems such as school and nursery a reality (Rehm and Bradley 2005). It was estimated that in 2001, 6000 children in the UK were thought to be reliant on some form of technology for their well-being and sometimes survival. In almost all cases, parents took on this technical aspect of their child's care and in doing so became expert parents, with varying support from CCN teams and the wider multidisciplinary network.

The support that can be offered by the CCN team can be in the form of information, technological training and education to provision of a short break or respite care to the family. Taking into account the complexity of the care demands of some of these children and the high level of skill and aptitude required to be able to safely care for the child, it is vital that the person providing the care has the appropriate level of expertise. Some children will receive the care of a robustly trained carer and some will require the enhanced clinical and assessment skills of a qualified nurse. All care provision will depend on a thorough holistic nursing assessment of need; decisions will then be made by a qualified specialist practitioner in CCN (CCNs with a degree in specialist practice) to establish who is the most appropriate health care professional to provide the care.

A proportion of CCN services also run nurse-led initiatives such as clinics for eczema and childhood constipation (such as the authors' CCN team). This way of working not only epitomises sound resource management but also responds to recommendations from *Liberating the Talents* (DH 2002), which suggested that nurses are in a prime position to lead health care in the community. This dynamic nurse-led service is usually led by senior, appropriately qualified clinical nurses, and although the role of the newly qualified nurses is limited in this arena, the opportunity for learning from expert and innovative nursing practice cannot be over-estimated.

This overview aims to demonstrate the complexity and diversity of the children cared for on this caseload and, in so doing, offers an insight into the opportunities available for a qualified nurse working in this arena.

Skill mix within the CCN team

With the drive to provide increasing amounts of care for children and young people in the community, nurse training seeks to prepare nurses to be 'fit for purpose' and 'fit for practice' in both hospital and community settings (UKCC 1999, NMC 2004). Since the introduction of the Project 2000 nurse training programme, pre-registration nurse training now includes significant component relating to community practice, which gives greater opportunities for nurses to practice in this arena once qualified (Hickey and Hardiman 2000). However, it could be argued that due to the need for greater autonomy and independence expected of a nurse working in the community and the lack of access to help and support that may be present in a more acute environment, the newly qualified practitioner does not have all the skills needed to take on all aspects of the role.

Proctor (1998) suggested that all nurses working with sick children in the community should have a specialist CCN qualification. However, it could be argued that not all CCN teams have access to local Specialist Practitioner programmes, and to enrol in such courses, there is an expectation that the applicant would have at least 1 year to 18 months experience working in the community. For stakeholders involved in strategically workforce planning, the option of employing newly qualified nurses in these roles may be attractive, with the expectation that the nurse will undertake the Specialist Practitioner Degree in CNN, thus developing the role and enhancing practice (Neill and Muir 1997, Proctor *et al.* 1999).

Traditionally, the CCN team has predominately consisted of senior, experienced children's nurses, with a community qualification/background (While and Dyson 2000). However, the development and expansion of such teams have implications for the service and recruitment of appropriately qualified staff. There are increasing opportunities for a less-experienced but qualified nurse to provide good quality, effective care, which is also cost effective and meets the needs of the children and their families (Jenkins-Clarke and Carr-Hill 2001). Indeed, within the authors' own CCN team, there has been a significant shift from a service staffed exclusively by senior (Band 6/7) nurses to a multidisciplinary team that currently employs a nursing workforce of Band 5 (2 WTE, Whote Time Equivalent), Band 6 (3.6 WTE) and Band 7 (1 WTE).

This in itself may raise new challenges and challenge ingrained working practices and encourage qualified CCNs to rethink their role and the role of junior colleagues. It can be difficult to define and quantify the role of a CCN and establish role differences between the grades of nursing staff, especially when skill mix is a new concept within the team.

Benner's (1984) seminal work on expertise in nursing practice provides an invaluable framework in supporting the differences between the roles. Benner (1984) demonstrated how subtle yet definite transitions throughout the nurse's career enable her to move from novice to expert depending on her ability to learn and progress. The five key stages are:

1. Novice (i.e. student nurse at the beginning of training parent or carer at the beginning of learning process).
2. Advanced beginner (i.e. student nurse nearing completion of training).
3. Competence (i.e. newly qualified nurse).
4. Proficient (i.e. experienced nurse).
5. Expert (advanced nursing practice) (Benner 1984).

This is a fluid process, and nurses may never reach the stage of expert or may flow between stages. Benner *et al.* (1996) demonstrated to us that clinical or technical nursing skills are a component of nursing care, which may be relatively simple to learn. There is often an expectation that parents and carers to become proficient in a range of high-tech clinical skills without having any formal nurse training. Parents will often become so competent in these skills, that they are the undisputed experts in the care of their child. However, when it comes to nursing, expertise is defined by the accumulation of subtle skills such as deep understanding of medical/nursing theory, intuition, knowing what needs to be achieved and exactly how to achieve it. It is hoped that a newly qualified nurse will be competent, able to plan and perform a task with minimal or no supervision. Meretoja *et al.* (2002) described that, at this stage of practice, a nurse should be able to offer holistic management rather than breaking care down in to tasks. For the newly qualified nurse in the CCN team, this stage can provoke some anxiety while the nurse moves to a more autonomous role without the comfort of immediate access to guidance from a more senior colleague. There is an expectation that newly qualified nurses will assume this autonomous role quickly and be able to go into children's homes and provide safe, high-quality care with no immediate supervision. This poses particular challenges in ensuring the safety of the child and family and also the safety of the newly qualified nurse without suppressing their abilities and undermining their practice.

Nursing assessments within the CCN team are performed by the key worker. Hallett and Pateman (2000) suggested that this can be a contentious issue for junior nurses who may be practiced at assessing very sick patients in an acute setting. Tensions may arise when junior nurses feel that they have the ability to produce a robust nursing assessment but are not enabled to do so. Nursing assessments of children who often have multiple and complex needs are based on the *Framework for the Assessment of Children in Need* (2000), ensuring that all aspects of the child and family's life and impact of illness or condition are considered. Many commissioning decisions are made on the strength of a robust nursing assessment; it is therefore felt that a skilled and qualified CCN is the professional in the best position to use her expert skills to complete these assessments.

Unclear role definition is not a new concept within primary care (Hallett and Pateman 2000). In response to this, alongside job descriptions and in accordance with the knowledge and skill framework, guidance was provided to simplify the expectations of each role (Table 5.1).

The reflective narrative that follows aims to demonstrate some of the dilemmas and proposed solutions and recommendations for practice are consequently suggested.

Amber Barnum, the co-author of this chapter, continues with her narrative around the development of her role and a reflection on a critical incident.

Table 5.1   Expectations of Band 5 and Bank 6 Community nurses

Role of the Band 6 CCN	Role of the Band 5 newly qualified community children's staff nurse
• Preceptor/role model • Caseload manager/dependency and workload planning • Key worker/care co-ordination • Nursing assessment • Source of information • Day-to-day clinical leadership • Provision of an on call service including palliative/end of life care • Personal and service development • Collaborative working • Teaching and training children, parents and carers • Developing and running nurse-led services • Extended nurse prescribing (where qualified) • Life-long learning	• Preceptee • Clinical work under the direction of the CCN • Co-worker • Deliver and evaluate care in accordance with care plans/guidelines/care pathways • Work under the direction of the CCN to provide an out of hours service • Personal development and involvement with service development • Teach and train children, parents and carers using competency packages developed by the CCN • Life-long learning, aim for commencement of CCN Specialist Practice Degree within 3 years

---

Background to take a post within the Children's Community Nursing Team

My pre-registration children's nurse training began within a general Paediatric ward; this remained my clinical base throughout my nursing course. My training involved many different ward settings, which led me into my third year where I spent 6 months within a CCN team. The CCN team was diverse, supportive and provided an appropriate amount of time to observe and learn about nursing children and their families within their own home. From this placement, I learnt that CCN was varied and different from any other role that I had experienced. I decided that this was the area that I ultimately wanted to specialise in, post-registration. Once I qualified, I decided that I needed to consolidate my clinical nursing skills. I spent 10 months on a general paediatric ward. During this time, I maintained contact with the local CCN team. I spent time with them, and this enabled me to introduce myself and become familiar with the way the team worked. A Band 5 post was advertised, and I applied with 10-month ward experience. I began my job as a Community Children's Staff Nurse with 12 months post-registration experience. After a 4-week structured induction, I visited children and their families autonomously in the community setting.

Case scenario using Gibbs reflective cycle (1988)

In this case scenario, I will reflect upon my interactions with a mother of a child who is severely disabled, using Gibbs (1988) reflective cycle. Issues that arose from this will be discussed and analysed with reference to supporting literature. Gibbs (1988) informed us that reflection takes place after an event. It is a series of processes, which are followed to gain a deeper understanding of the event that took place. There are five stages to this process; they are description of the event, feelings, identified evaluation, analysis and conclusion followed with an action plan.

Stage 1: Description of the event

The child and mother at the core of this scenario will be given pseudonyms. The child will be known as Harry, his mother (a single parent) will be known as Clare, their confidentiality will be maintained at all times in accordance with the Nursing and Midwifery Council (NMC 2004, section 5.1, p. 8).

Harry was 12 years old and he had been developing normally until tragically he was involved in a road traffic accident, while on holiday, in which he sustained a severe brain injury. Harry was subsequently intubated, ventilated and transferred to a paediatric intensive care unit (PICU). Harry's mother was told the sad news by the PICU consultant that her son had severe, irreversible brain damage, and it was understood that he was unlikely to survive post-extubation. The PICU registrar discussed with Clare the options that were available to them post-extubation; Clare was informed about her local children's hospice or alternatively should she so wish, she could take Harry home for end of life care, with the support from the multidisciplinary team (including CCN team). Clare decided that she would prefer Harry to be cared for in the acute children's ward in the tertiary centre as she felt that she had built up relationships with the doctors and nurses and wished to remain there at this sensitive time. The PICU registrar liaised with the children's ward and organised for Harry's immediate transfer. Against all the odds, Harry survived and had a 4-month stay in the children's ward. Subsequently, it was decided that Harry was not, as had been believed, at the end of his life, and plans were commenced to get Harry home. Clare met with the multidisciplinary team to plan his future care, and it was decided that Harry should return home as soon as equipment and supplies could be organised. Harry was extremely disabled and would need 24-hour care to meet his needs, which Clare was determined to provide. The family home needed significant adaptations to meet Harry's moving and handling needs, but this would take several months of organisation before this could be achieved. Clare decided to forge ahead, with the aim of getting Harry home as soon as possible. Harry was discharged home after adequate plans were made, equipment and supplies were procured and in place. During the first 2 weeks of Harry being at home, Clare expressed to the CCN that it was challenging managing Harry's needs but she were coping, with the help of friends and family and she did not wish for external support.

The senior CCN allocated to me Harry's routine gastrostomy change that day. It was the first time that it had been changed at home, and Clare had requested that I changed the tube and talked her through the process. I felt competent to undertake this procedure. This visit was identified as straightforward and was deemed appropriate for me to manage. When I arrived, Clare was very emotional and obviously under immense strain. She confided in me that she was finding it very difficult to cope with her son, and she expressed that she felt desperate and suicidal. Clare was extremely frightened of what she might do if she was left alone. I reassured Clare that I would not leave her and Harry alone and continued to listen, while letting the CCN team know the sequence of events that were taking place and discussing a plan of action for the family. I asked Clare whether there was any one she felt comfortable with that she wanted present while we continued to discuss her stress, concerns and ensure Harry's safety. Clare explained that she would not mind if her sister were present. I contacted Clare's sister and explained the circumstances and asked whether it would be possible for her to come and sit with Clare and Harry while we continued our discussion and made arrangements. Clare's sister promptly arrived at the family's home. I explained that I needed to return back to the office to discuss Clare's concerns with the team. I then requested that Clare's sister would remain present with her sister and niece while alternative plans were made. Clare's sister agreed that she would stay within the family home until alternative plans were made.

I immediately contacted my team manager from my car and explained the circumstances. I returned to the office and contacted Harry's local social worker and paediatrician, and with Clare's permission, I requested a home visit from her GP. I spoke to the local Social Services Respite Care Centre to see whether they could accommodate Harry immediately, which they could. It was decided in partnership with Clare that Harry would be admitted to the local Social Services Respite Care Centre while alternative care arrangements could be made. Harry arrived at the Respite Care Centre in the interim, 4 hours from the start of my visit until more robust plans were made.

Stage 2: Feelings

I found this situation incredibly daunting, Clare's distress and anxiety was evident, and it was very difficult to calm her down and dissolve the situation. I felt very concerned about Clare's safety, which of course would have a profound impact on Harry. I had never dealt with a situation like this. I was very anxious about not saying and doing the right things in this situation as any action on my part may make the situation worse. I endeavoured to ensure that I maintain their safety at all times, and in conjunction with this, I reassured Clare that I would ensure that she was not left alone with Harry. I had to think on my feet, rapidly and logically under immense pressure while also listening and reassuring Clare. I also had to try to maintain a calm atmosphere. I felt overwhelmed by the fact that I was not in my comfort zone and also that I was a guest in their home. I was also concerned that I was alone and there were no senior members of the team to immediately consult with or witness what I was hearing, observing and communicating. I felt extremely vulnerable. I was conscious of my lack of experience and wanted to ensure that I maintained open clear honest communication with Clare, while adequately protecting Harry. I did not want to make plans about what the next step was until I had spoken to the team; however, I was aware of my duty to ensure both Harry and Clare were safe.

Stage 3: Evaluation

The incident had positive and negative outcomes. I ensured that Harry and his mother were safe at all times, Harry's safety and well-being being my main priority. As a result of this critical incident, Clare was able to identify that to have Harry at home she would need a lot of support from professional bodies to work in partnership with Clare and her family. I was encouraged and supported by the team to inform Harry's paediatrician and social services to devise a plan of action for Harry and Clare. I was empowered by the CCN team to continue liaising with Clare and the wider multidisciplinary team, to come up with a workable solution. It is satisfying to know that the team was able to support and encourage my professional decision making in this situation, while offering their guidance and expertise. Another positive outcome was that Clare was then able to access counselling and emergency mental health support while Harry's was being cared for in a safe environment.

There were, however, two negative outcomes of this scenario, which I have identified. I felt unprepared for this type of situation; I was very inexperienced in the community and was not sure how the multidisciplinary teams worked or what resources were locally available. I knew of the Respite Care Facility but was unsure of their eligibility criteria and remit. I was aware that if I had the knowledge of the wider multi-professional teams, I could reassure Clare about appropriate actions to take and how Harry's subsequent care would be managed. At the time, I was aware that I felt very overwhelmed by my responsibilities, and this, in turn, affected my practice after the incident. Although the event had a positive result, I did feel that my confidence had been affected. I felt that if I was unprepared for that situation, what else was I unprepared for? I needed a lot of support and clinical supervision following the incident to help me learn from this and move on. I also found that I had to learn about boundary setting. I wanted to visit Harry every day to check whether things were OK but I was aware that this was not productive for myself and most importantly Harry and Clare. However, I could not distinguish what was too much or too little support and intervention at this time.

Stage 4: Analysis

It is important to remember that the team could not have been able to predict that this scenario was going to happen. Recognising the unpredictability of CCN is imperative. In my experience, it is essential to utilise the team's expertise and ensure that you are aware of how to seek advice while managing stressful, complex needs of families. Identifying limitations and recognising the need to manage a family's care with a more experienced colleague is crucial when practising as a newly qualified nurse.

Hickey (2000) investigated what jobs newly qualified nurses sought post-qualification. The findings suggest that there were three contributory factors that affected the newly qualified nurses' decision to work (or not) in the community. They were identified as a lack of interest in community nursing, feeling unprepared and wanting to consolidate their learning before working within the community.

In my experience, it was very important that I spent almost a year on a paediatric ward before entering the community setting. I felt that it was essential to consolidate my nursing skills in a safe environment with immediate access to nursing and medical support. Hickey and Hardiman (2000) explained that newly qualified nurses have expressed that they did not feel fully prepared to work in a community setting without first consolidating their nursing skills in a hospital environment, finding the stringent support systems beneficial. Through my analysis, I have identified that it is important that newly qualified members of the community team should have a robust induction, and autonomous visiting should not take place too early.

Stage 5: Action plan

The outcome of this scenario resulted in this team identifying a key worker and co-worker system. Although a key worker system was already in operation, my role was not clearly defined. This initiative encouraged good communication within the team and allowed junior staff to have a key worker to liaise with and be guided by. Patient allocation practices also changed as it was identified that all children on the caseload require a key worker and that junior members of the team would support the CCN by working as a co-worker. This system has proven to be very effective. It has enabled the junior members of the team to be empowered and more certain of their role. A CCN within the team has taken on the role of preceptor to help me to maximise my learning experience and therefore improve my practice. It has been identified within the team that I was able to visit on my own too quickly after recruitment, and in response to this a more robust induction system is being developed to ensure that future members of the team follow a clear set of guidelines and competencies to support them in their new role. I have learnt a lot about my professional boundaries, clinical skills and limitations within the community. I feel that CCN offers an individual child and family focused approach to health care, and I am very privileged and proud to work within a CCN team.

Lucy Edwards continues:

Reflection on the above account

It is evident from this insightful reflective narrative that role clarity and support systems were sub-optimal at this time. The sheer unpredictability and diversity that makes CCN practice so challenging can also present newly qualified staff with difficult and demanding situations. Kramer (1974) described the phenomenon of 'reality shock', whereby newly qualified nurses who thought they were prepared for becoming a staff nurse have an experience that severely undermines them and confirms that they are not fully prepared for their new role, which is evident in this reflection. The result of this critical incident caused the CCN team to develop new ways of working and embracing the new concept of skill mix within the team. Once clear role expectations were established, it became evident that to improve both working practices, thus improving the experience for the newly qualified staff nurse, a key worker (senior CCN) supported by a co-worker (newly qualified nurse) system may prove successful.

Families have repeatedly identified that they would benefit from a key worker, who will be responsible for orchestrating their child's care and be their first point of contact (Mukherjee *et al.* 1999, ACT 2003, Sloper *et al.* 2006). The key worker system has elements of preceptorship, in that the junior nurse will be supported and guided for each patient and time was set aside each day to reflect on the day's activities.

Formal clinical supervision sessions were also organised. The advantages of this initiative were manifold. The CCN offered leadership, support and acted as a role model, enabling the junior nurse to consolidate her skills and move on to the next phase of learning. Both parties gained an insight into their strengths and limitations by sharing knowledge and experiences. A robust orientation

Table 5.2 Newly qualified staff nurse orientation timeline of events

Timeframe	Expected achievement
Week 1–2	Trust induction
	Mandatory training
Weeks 2–12	Meet with preceptor weekly to discuss/reflect upon experiences including the allocation of a clinical supervisor
	Discuss boundary setting and lone working policy with preceptor
	Shadow all team members, resulting in an understanding of roles
	Organise visits with the teams and agencies with which the CCN team work collaboratively, i.e. Children's Hospice, Child Development Centre, Acute Children's Wards, Social Services, Children's Disability Teams, Voluntary Services, Special Schools
	Attend Nurse-Led Clinics
	Observe in Practice:
	• Hospital discharge procedures
	• Admission to CCN team procedure
	• Assessment of children and their families who have acute needs
	• Assessment of children and their families who have complex needs
	• Various clinical procedures performed at home such as administration of intravenous medication, home oxygen, home ventilation, wound dressings, home traction
	• Respite allocation panel
	Become competent in a range of clinical skills using current training packages and trust policies and procedures
Weeks 12–26	Begin to work autonomously in children's homes, recognising limitations and with robust support from preceptor/CCN team
	Monthly clinical supervision
	Keep practice portfolio
Weeks 26–52	Continue to work within scope of professional practice with continued but decreasing support from preceptor/CCN team
	Undertake an appraisal and set objectives for the following year.

package was designed (Table 5.2) and will be piloted in due course outlining a more realistic timeline of events expected of the newly appointed staff nurse. Timeframes are flexible to respond to part-time working and individual learning need. This incorporated the development and updating of clinical guidelines, protocols and care pathways to guide practice.

Boundary setting was highlighted as an issue for development. CCNs are in a unique position in their role. The shift of power in favour of the family is evident in the community. CCNs are guests in the home of the child and family which in itself can be confusing and compromising for a less-experienced nurse. Suddenly the boundaries can become blurred, and what is a professional relationship can seem very friendly. According to Samwell (2005), CCNs require exceptional insight and interpersonal skills to manage these frequently intense relationships with families and the nurse must ask herself, 'Who am I doing this for?' What is, at best, a truly empowering relationship is in danger of becoming a dependent, disempowered partnership. Acknowledging that these can be pitfalls and potential hazards in CCN allows us to pre-empt situations and make positive steps towards fostering a therapeutic, professional relationship.

Future learning needs were also identified by developing a personal development plan. Education is given high priority, and junior nurses are encouraged to undertake a post-graduate degree programme in Specialist Practice in CCN within the 3 years of their appointment to the team. This offers an excellent opportunity to consolidate the nurse's experience and begin to make the transition towards expert practice.

Conclusion

This is an exciting time in CCN. After years of having a low profile, many CCN teams are able to reap the rewards of years of determined effort in promoting the development of services to meet the ever-changing needs of local populations. The concept of incorporating newly qualified nurses into an established and experienced team has been a challenge. It has not been without difficulties, but working practices and team working have evolved and improved as a result. The drive continues to care for children at home or in the community wherever possible, and the standards stipulated by the National Service Frameworks Department for Education and skills and, Department of Health London (2004) support the work of CCN teams and encourage innovative and responsive practice. Children are being discharged from hospital earlier or bypass acute care services altogether. The key to CCN services success has been to provide a service that children and families really want, in a timely and flexible manner. To sustain this level of innovation and support, CCNs need to look towards inspiring newly qualified nurses with the passion that has brought CCN services this far, providing children and their families with highly motivated, dedicated and skilled nurses.

References

Association for Children with Life Threatening or Terminal Conditions and Their Families (ACT) (2003). *Assessment of Children with Life-Limiting Conditions and Their Families. A Guide to Effective Care Planning*. Bristol: ACT.

Benner P (1984). *From Novice to Expert. Excellence and Power in Clinical Nursing Practice*. Menlo Park: Addison Wesley.

Benner P, Tanner CA and Chesla CA (1996). *Expertise in Nursing Practice. Caring, Clinical Judgement and Ethics.* New York: Springer Publishing.

Cramp C, Hughes N and Dale G (2003). Children's home nursing: Results of a national survey. *Paediatric Nursing*, 15(8), 40–43.

Department for Education and Skills (DfES) and Department of Health (DH) (2004). *National Service Framework for Children, Young People and Maternity Services: Children and Young People Who are Ill.* London: DH.

Department of Health (DH) (2002). *Liberating the Talents.* London: DH.

Department of Health and Department for Education and Employment (2000). Framework for the Assessment of Children in Need and Their Families. London: The Stationery Office.

Drew J, Nathan D and Hall D (2002). Role of a paediatric nurse in primary care 1: Research issues. *British Journal of Nursing*, 11(22), 1452–1460.

Gibbs G (1988). *Learning by Doing. A Guide to Teaching and Learning Methods.* Oxford: Brookes University.

Eaton N (2001). Models of community children's nursing. *Paediatric Nursing*, 13(1), 32–36.

English National Board for Nursing, Midwifery and Health Visiting (ENB) and Department of Health (DH) (1999). *Sharing the Care: Resource Pack to Support Diana, Princess of Wales Community Children's Nursing Teams.* London: ENB.

Hallett CE and Pateman BD (2000). The 'invisible assessment' the role of the staff nurse in the community setting. *Journal of Clinical Nursing*, 9, 751–762.

Hickey G (2000). Newly qualified and into the community? *Paediatric Nursing*, 12(9), 30–32.

Hickey G and Hardiman R (2000). Using questionnaires to ask nurses about working in the community: Problems of definition. *Health and Social Care in the Community*, 8(1), 70–73.

House of Commons Health Committee (1997). *Health Services for Children and Young People in the Community: Home and School. Third Report.* London: The Stationery Office.

Jenkins-Clarke S and Carr-Hill R (2001). Changes, challenges and choices for the primary health care workforce: Looking to the future. *Journal of Advanced Nursing*, 34(6), 842–849.

Kramer M (1974). *Reality Shock. Why Nurses Leave Nursing.* St Louis: Mosby.

Meretoja R, Eriksson E and Leino-Kilpi H (2002). Indicators for competent nursing practice. *Journal of Nursing Management*, 10, 95–102.

Ministry of Health (1959). *The Welfare of Children in Hospital – Report of the Committee (Chairman Sir H Platt).* London: HMSO.

Mountford S, Widdas D and Linter S (2005). A 'new' national health service. In: Sidey A and Widdas D (eds), *Textbook of Community Children's Nursing*, Chapter 3. London: Elsevier.

Mukherjee S, Beresford B and Sloper P (1999). *Unlocking Key Working.* Bristol: Policy Press.

National Health Service (NHS) Executive (1996). *Child Health in the Community. A Guide to Good Practice.* London: The Stationery Office.

Neill SJ and Muir J (1997). Educating the new community children's nurses: Challenges and opportunities. *Nurse Education Today*, 17, 8–10.

New Opportunities Fund (NOF) (2002). *Palliative Care for Children Programme: Guidance Notes.* London: NOF.

Nursing and Midwifery Council (NMC) (2004). *Code of Professional Conduct. Standards for Conduct Performance and Ethics.* London: NMC.

Proctor S, Campbell S, Biott C, Edward S, Moran M, Redapath N and Steljes J (1998). *Preparation for the Developing Role of the Community Children's Nurse.* London: English National Board for Nursing, Midwifery and Health Visiting.

Rehm RS and Bradley JF (2005). Normalization of families raising a child who is medically fragile/technology dependent and developmentally delayed. *Qualitative Health Research*, 15(6), 807–820.

Royal College of Nursing (RCN) (2004). *Directory of Community Children's Nursing Services*, 16th edn. London: RCN.

Samwell B (2005). Nursing the family and supporting the nurse: Exploring the nurse–patient relationship in community children's nursing. In: Sidey A and Widdas D (eds), *Textbook of Community Children's Nursing*, Chapter 11. London: Elsevier.

Sloper P, Greco V, Beecham J and Webb R (2006). Key worker services for disabled children: What characteristics of services lead to better outcomes for children and families? *Child: Care, Health and Development*, 32(2), 147–157.

Tatman M and Jones S (2005). Issues for the composition of community children's nursing teams. In: Sidey A and Widdas D (eds). *Textbook of Community Children's Nursing*, Chapter 16. London: Elsevier.

United Kingdom Central Council for Nursing, Midwifery and Health Visiting (UKCC) (1999). *Fitness for Practice*. London: UKCC.

Wagner J, Power EJ, Fox (1988). *Technology dependent children: Hospital versus home care.* Office of Technology Assessment Task Force. Philadelphia: Lippincott.

While AC and Dyson L (2000). Characteristics of paediatric home care provision: The two dominant models in England. *Child: Care, Health and Development*, 26(4), 263–276.

Whiting M (1998). Expanding community children's nursing services. *British Journal of Community Nursing*, 3(4), 183–184.

Chapter 6

The Public Health Practitioner

Janice Christie, Jackie Parkes and Jayne Price

Introduction

The aim of this chapter is to stimulate debate among children's nurses about current and future roles in relation to public health. There are many types of practitioners working in public health, but few people can describe themselves as public health practitioners. There is considerable discussion in the literature about what constitutes a public health nurse and public health nursing and exactly what contribution nurses make to public health. In this chapter, we will consider the role of public health in relation to children's nurses, primarily. This will include a discussion of public health issues that encompass all nurses and all activities aimed at protecting and improving the health of *populations* of children, young people and their families. The role of the children's nurse has been described as '...carer, health educator, health promoter, the researcher, empowerer and the advocate' (Ross 2003, p. 37). Although it is unlikely that any one children's nurse can hope to be expert in all areas, children's nurses have a contribution to make to each area with the possibility of specialising in one or two. In this chapter, we give three examples of how children's nurses can work to improve child public health. These examples include accounts from a staff nurse, a health visitor and a nurse researcher.

In the UK, there are ~12 million children and young people under the age of 16 who comprise ~20% of the population (ONS 2002). This proportion has been decreasing over the past 40 years (from 25% in 1971 to 19% in 2004 in England and Wales) due to declining fertility rates (ONS 2002). Although it is important to remember that most children and young people develop 'normally' and are 'well' and remain so for most of their childhood and adolescence, the social contexts in which they live and therefore the factors influencing their health have changed. The modern day epidemics affecting child health include obesity, diabetes, heart disease and behavioural problems which require interventions at the level of individual, community and nationally. Although few children in the developed world could be considered to live in absolute poverty, there is now recognition that many live in relative poverty with the gap between the rich and the poor widening and giving rise to social inequalities in health (Black *et al.* 1980).

There are ~1.5 billion children in the world and 85% of them live in developing countries (Blair *et al.* 2003). Therefore, it is not sufficient for children's nurses to be complacent and think of 'community' in local or national terms only, since modern international travel increases transmission rates between countries (Wilson 1995). This was exemplified by the SARS outbreak in 2003 and concerns regarding a potential bird flu (H5NI) pandemic (Bartlett and Hayden 2005). As a public health practitioner, awareness of the global issues affecting child health in developing countries is increasingly coming to our attention.

Children's nurses must understand that they have a part to play in lobbying governments, drug companies and supporting charities for more and better child public health initiatives to help combat malaria, treat AIDS and support orphaned children, prevent malnutrition and promote better maternal and infant health. A more detailed discussion of these issues is beyond the scope of this chapter, but an excellent introduction to the topic of global child health is provided by Blair and colleagues (2003, Chapter 2).

What is public health?

The Faculty of Public Health (2008) summarised the key components of the public health approach, which includes four key points that it (1) is population based; (2) emphasises collective responsibility for health, its protection and disease prevention; (3) recognises the key role of the state, linked to a concern for the underlying socio-economic and wider determinants of health, as well as disease and (4) emphasises partnerships with all those who contribute to the health of the population. These components relate to the conceptualisation of modern public health practices as 'everyone's business'.

Possibly, the most commonly cited definition of public health was quoted by Sir Donald Acheson (DH 1988), which was derived from Winslow, a professor of Public Health at Yale University in 1920:

> Public health is the science and art of preventing disease, prolonging life and promoting health through organised efforts of society (p. 1).

This definition, while emphasising biological health outcomes, hints at the breadth of effort that can be undertaken to achieve public health. A more detailed definition is provided by Blair *et al.* (2003) who specifically define child public health as:

> the study of patterns of health and illness in children and young people, the various factors which affect their health, and ways in which we – as individuals, organizations, professions, and societies – can modify these factors in order to improve the health and well-being of all young people (p. 2).

This definition underlines the importance of evidence-based working in public health in both undertaking assessment and meeting needs for groups of people.

The broad aim of child public health is to help children and young people achieve and maintain their health through disease prevention (e.g. immunisation), health promotion (e.g. healthy eating) and empowerment (e.g. making informed choices). In the UK, the majority of 'well-child care' or prevention is provided by primary care services – the general practitioner (GP) and community nursing services – mainly the health visitor (also known as Specialist Community Public Health Nurses), although there is little research evidence available about the effectiveness of well-child care models (Dinkevich *et al.* 2001). Brocklehurst (2004) has urged nurses to incorporate 'a public health perspective' in their work as a means of providing a broader and more strategic way of thinking about patient care. Indeed, the Nursing Midwifery Council (NMC) clearly specifies that nurses have a professional responsibility to 'protect and support health of individuals and *the wider community*' (NMC 2004, p. 4). For the children's nurse, this would mean adopting a more strategic approach to the health of the community in which children are living, understanding more about the factors that directly and indirectly influence child health in that community and acting in collaboration with other professionals to influence the determinants of child health through protection, health promotion or disease prevention.

Why public health?

History

Ideas of health promotion and environmental action described within our definitions of public health can be identified within ancient societies (Rosen 1993). Four thousand years ago, cities on the Indian subcontinent had developed environmental sanitation programmes that included the use of underground drains and public baths. Greek and Roman civilisations drawing on the work of Hippocrates and Galen featured prevention through use of diet and exercise to maintain and restore health. These ideas were later revived by the 18th century European doctors.

The development of modern public health practice was also dependent on other historical developments. Changes in political philosophy have influenced public health (Porter 1999). Revolutions in America and France asserted rights to freedom and well-being for all citizens. During the industrial revolution, people migrated to cities to gain work as the population density grew in urban environments and old sanitation systems became inadequate. Infection disease caused a high, preventable infant and child mortality rate from diarrhoea, measles, whooping cough, diphtheria, tuberculosis, cholera and smallpox. With more humanitarian social attitudes, particularly in relation to poor women and children (Blair *et al.* 2003), this brought about the rise of the sanitary movement in the 18th century. Environmental improvements in water supplies, sewage systems and development of vaccines against infections brought about major decreases in child mortality.

Broadly speaking, this approach later developed into preventive medicine (1900s) and then more recently (2000s) into the social model of disease with an emphasis on public policy and intersectoral working among health, social care, housing, transport and education (Pomerleau and McKee 2005). By the middle of the 20th century, there had been dramatic reductions in infectious diseases, resulting in longer life expectancy and increase in affluence. These social trends resulted in new patterns of chronic and lifestyle diseases in western societies. Health services have responded to these by a growing emphasis on maximising and promoting well-being, focusing on health rather than disease. The increasing survival rate of children with complex health needs from once fatal illnesses has offered a challenge to children's nursing. Such children, although often technology dependent, require multi-professional support to families in home-based rather than hospital-based services (Hughes and Horsburgh 2002). The move towards family-focused care within the community settings has increased the potential for children's nurses to adopt collectivist, public health thinking in everyday practice.

There is not scope to review the historical developments of public health in more detail here, but Professor Warren has provided a fascinating and in-depth account entitled 'A Chronology of State Medicine, Public Health, Welfare and Related Services in Britain 1066–1999' (Warren 2000).

Changes in child health

Enormous strides have been made in child health in the past 100 years: many common, lethal infections have been eradicated (small pox), malnutrition is seldom seen and perinatal and infant mortality continues to decline. With social change have come new challenges including health risk behaviours (teenage pregnancy, illicit drug taking, smoking and obesity) and mental health problems.

Ironically, changes in medical technology have contributed to the 'burden' of disease and disability in our society (Stewart-Brown 2002) by improving survival for children with life-limiting or debilitating conditions such as cystic fibrosis, childhood cancers and complex disability. Furthermore, with improved awareness and diagnosis and shifting social patterns, there is an apparent increase in the numbers of children experiencing behavioural and learning problems and increases in the prevalence of conditions such as autism, attention deficit and hyperactivity disorders. All of these are likely to be relatively rare conditions but requiring high intensity use of health and social care services with public health and clinical strategies to help ensure the best possible outcomes.

Determinants of child health

Child and young person's health is one of the most important areas of public health. Blair *et al.* (2003) proposed two important reasons for the underlying importance of child public health. First, that all children have a right to lead as healthy and enjoyable a life as possible, free from disease and stress as far as possible, and this has been ratified globally in the United Nations (1989) 'Convention on the Rights of the Child'. To this end alone, pursuing child public health as a strategy to help ensure the rights of the child are protected is essential. Second, that the children of today are our collective future, and investing in and protecting their health is vitally important to help them achieve the best possible physical, psychological and social outcomes.

The key determinants of child health have been summarised as including poverty and income inequality, families and relationships; nutrition; physical and social environment; social attitudes and stigma; risk-taking behaviours; genetics and health service provision (Blair *et al.* 2003). The 'life-course approach' that has been described in relation to chronic disease (Kuh and Ben-Shlomo 1997) suggests that health later on in adult life is largely determined by an interplay of early exposures and risk factors in infancy and childhood. The risk factors may be biological and include genetic predisposition to certain diseases (e.g. cancer), social including attitudes that underpin health behaviours (e.g. smoking, nutrition and sexual health) and/or economy that may influence choices and access to health care.

This suggests that the health and disease children experience have implications for their future well-being and even the future well-being of their children. This position highlights the importance of intervening early at every opportunity to influence the determinants of child health such as nutrition, exercise and parenting skills – helping parents to make informed choices, act as role models for their children and provide emotionally secure environments.

All nurses can influence public health through involvement in helping individuals make healthy decisions that will meet national goals for a more healthy society (DH 2004). Children's nurses have the opportunity to assist families and children to make healthy choices early in the lifespan when there is the potential for a full lifetime of benefit from interventions. Holman (1992) reviewed the development of 'public health thinking' and suggested a taxonomy of public health movements: health protection, disease prevention, health education/promotion, healthy public policy and community empowerment. We will use these headings to structure our discussion on children's nurses' public health roles.

Health protection

Health protection is characterised by the regulation of human behaviour to protect the health of citizens. Examples of health protection measures are fluoridisation of water supplies and recent child booster seat legislation. The approach has been criticised because it stresses collectivist ideals rather than individual autonomy (the individual's right to make healthy choices for themselves).

Disease prevention

Caplan (1961) identified three categories of prevention: primary prevention relating to the maintenance of health, secondary prevention corresponding to early detection of disease and tertiary prevention concerning containing and limiting the effects of a condition. Traditionally, 'prevention' is associated with medical activity that aims to reduce morbidity and early mortality. Examples of primary prevention-orientated interventions are immunisation programmes that aim to stop people developing infectious disease. Secondary prevention often involves the screening and intervention targeted at individuals or groups at high risk. For screening to be effective, however, it must meet rigorous criteria regarding the disease or health problem, the test, follow up and treatment and economic resources (Robinson and Elkan 1996).

When formal programmes of Child Health Surveillance were introduced in the UK, during the late 1980s, they were based on the ideas of early detection and remedial action for childhood illness and disability (Hall 1989, Butler 1989). As children reached specified ages, the well-being of children was checked by doctors, school nurses and health visitors. Centralised records were kept of the results of these assessments. Owing to growing research evidence regarding the ineffectiveness of such programmes, the current emphasis has changed to a core health promotion programme with additional services targeted at those most at risk (Hall and Elliman 2003).

Health education/promotion

Health education is the provision of learning experiences to enable people to change their behaviours and habits to improve their present or future health (Naidoo and Wills 1994). The approach assumes that individuals have the ability to change their own health status. However, this is a simplistic assumption and ignores the complex relationship between behaviour, social change and environmental factors. As a health education approach emphasises the individual, it can potentially lead to 'victim blaming' and be used as a political rationale for not engaging with collective public policies. The concept has developed into health promotion in which the role of the health professional is that of a facilitator or 'empowerer' of health. Health promotion helps make a 'healthy choice an easy choice' (Tones and Green 2004); therefore, it includes efforts to tackle social and environmental causes of health. An example of health education is when a nurse gives a father of a child with a chest infection information about the effect that smoking is having on his child's health. Health promotion occurs when a nurse teaches a group of teenage mothers attending a mother and toddler group cooking skills emphasising healthy eating and five portions of fruit and vegetables per day.

Healthy public policy

The aim of 'healthy public policy' is to create a social, economic and physical environment that helps people make healthy choices. This approach derives from concern about the impact of poverty on health and is aligned with the Ottawa Charter (World Health Organisation 1986). Until recently, much of the public health work undertaken by the National Health Service (NHS) involved an individualist focus that failed to recognise the importance of social groups such as families and communities. The Healthy City and Healthy School movements co-ordinated by World Health Organisation (WHO) are examples of this type of work in which emphasis is placed on creating healthy environments through engaging a multi-agency approach that integrates the work of organisations that are outside health services. Within the UK, Health Improvement Plans, Health Action Zones (Department of Health Social Services and Public Safety 2002, DH 1999b) and Sure Start (Ministerial Group on the Family 1998) are further examples of public healthy policy. Critics of the approach have raised concerns that it is not practical or effective and that it creates a cultural climate in which the system alone is responsible for ill-health.

Community empowerment

The concept of community empowerment concerns local groups of people participating in decision making regarding health, ideas that have international importance (WHO 1998). The right of people to participate in health care is defined in the WHO Alma-Ata statement (WHO 1978). Many of the recommendations from the Acheson report (DH 1998), which aimed to reduce inequalities in health, had a community or population focus. The ideology of community empowerment is rooted in collective action for local social and environmental justice (Ledwith 2005). Since it aims to increase the power and influence of disadvantaged groups (such as workers, women and ethnic minorities), it is a way allowing social excluded or marginalised groups of people in society (traveller families or the homeless) becoming included in decision making about their health. There is little emphasis on professional expertise in this approach. Critics state that the local and lay emphasis can lead to inadequately informed decision making and that it causes a piecemeal approach that hinders any major social or national reform. An example of community empowerment occurs when a nurse encourages disadvantaged mothers in a housing development beside a major road, to campaign the local council for safe play facilities.

Who is the public health practitioner in nursing?

This is something of an ongoing debate, especially given overlap between community nursing, primary care nursing and public health nursing. The WHO (2000) proposed a curriculum for a family health nurse, who was a care provider, community leader and manager. The concept of such a skilled, generalist nursing role based on family holistic and preventative care was proposed by and piloted by the Scottish Executive (2001, 2006). Throughout the UK, 'public health nurse' is often used almost as an 'umbrella term' to encompass activities by nurses aimed at the health of the community or population. It is often considered to be the remit of the health visitor and school nurse, mainly due to these professionals emphasis on prevention and health promotion.

The main roles of the school nurse have been identified as routine screening and surveillance, safe guarding health and welfare of children, a confidential advice service for young people, family support and health promotion (Hall 1999). Health visitors have a wide health promotion remit that range from assessing individual and community health to empowering good well-being choices, facilitating healthy action and influencing well-being policy (Council for the Education and Training of Health Visitors 1977). Craig (2000) therefore asked whether health visiting is perhaps just one of the many branches of nursing that contributes to public health or is public health just one of the many activities undertaken by health visitors? A study by Poulton *et al.* (2000) found that health visitors were more involved in collective forms of public health such as community empowerment and healthy public policy than other types of community nurses. Yet, Smith (2004) identified that health visitors were constrained to offer predominately family-focused care, delivering health promotion to mostly mothers and pre-school children. Policy documents in the UK have emphasised that health visitors have a family-centred public health role (DH 1999a, 2001).

The Chief Medical Officer (DH 2007) identified three broad categories of employees who through everyday activities influence public health:

- Workers who can help improve health and reduce social inequalities for example teachers, local business leaders, managers, social workers, housing officers, doctors and nurses.
- Professionals who spend much of their working time engaged in public health practices. Such professionals may work with groups and communities or individuals for example health visitors, environmental health officers and community development workers.
- People employed as public health specialists or senior managers who work across organisational boundaries or initiate and lead public health strategy or programmes.

The ideal of public health practice is targeting interventions (be it prevention, promotion, screening and policy) at the level of community or defined populations of people rather than the individual. A census study reviewing the components of public health practices undertaken by community nurses in Northern Ireland identified that most current activities centred on health education and preventative care for individual clients/patients rather than community-based groups although this study had a poor response rate (23%) (Poulton *et al.* 2000). Respondents felt that they needed more knowledge, skills and organisational support to undertake newer public health roles that involve collaboration with other agencies and political action.

Another part of the debate is that nurses contribute to public health in a very 'generalist' way and not as experts or strategists involved in directly assessing population need, estimating prevalence and survival, projecting future numbers and needs. Yet, others have argued that as nurses are based in the community, they are best placed to influence the health of the community (Hayes 2005). Regardless of which perspective most accurately conveys nursing, it is important that children's nurses appreciate how their public health role could be enhanced through further training, better identification of community-based opportunities for them to get involved with and through forming nursing networks and intersectoral collaborations. An example of the sorts of ways a hospital-based staff nurse working with children can influence child public health is described in Box 6.1.

Box 6.1 A day in the life of a children's staff nurse

As a staff nurse in acute children's ward in a district general hospital, everyday is varied, and my role obviously includes delivering physical care and other diverse roles such as teacher, facilitator, supporter, advocate and health promoter. The ward has medical and surgical beds; in addition, there are four infectious diseases cubicles.

Today is a typical day with a lot happening. This morning, I am in charge of the ward and assigned to care for two children with medical problems. Also, I have a third year nursing student working alongside me. In bed 1, we have a 2-year-old girl with a history of constipation; she has been commenced on medication and is being closely monitored. An integral part of her care is educating her parents on various aspects of managing constipation but also prevention. This includes ensuring a good fluid intake, a diet rich in fresh fruit and vegetables and administration/compliance of the appropriate medication (including safe storage). I liaise with the dietician who is also involved in this child's care. As this child is soon to be discharged, we must ensure good communication with the health visitor, community children's nurse (CCN) and GP who will continue to support the child and family after discharge. In the next bed, we have an 8-year-old boy who has been admitted with exacerbation of severe asthma. He requires regular nebulisers, review of his medication and much reassurance. His parents are both smokers and again education and support is required in this case.

This afternoon, I am helping to run a Well Teddy Clinic with the play specialist and a few of the other staff nurses and the student. These clinics occur on a regular basis with children from local primary schools, the aim being to use their teddy bear to educate them about hospitals, alleviate any fears about admission to hospital and in addition to provoke discussion about hospitals and child health issues. This session has a class of 28 children aged between 6 and 7. They arrive with their teacher, each clutching their teddy bear. Some of the teddies have bandages on their heads, others have plasters on their legs – the type of injuries or illnesses suffered by the teddies generate discussion with the children. They are shown around the hospital and are given the opportunity to play with a range of toys – stethoscopes, hospital jigsaws and dressing up clothes. We show them an X-ray where a child has ingested a 50 pence piece and then discuss the safety issues and the problems of putting small items in your mouth. One of the little girls says her teddy has a sore tummy as he ate too many sweets; this opens up the opportunity for talking with all the children about healthy eating. One of the other teddies has a bandage on its head, and the boy who owns it explains that it fell of his bicycle and hurt his head. This stimulates a discussion about the importance of wearing helmets when riding a bicycle. Initially, on arrival to the hospital, the class appeared very quiet and a bit hesitant; by the end of the session, they are interacting, asking questions, talking about health and illness and generally much more at ease in the hospital environment.

Today has been extremely busy; I have been managing the unit, teaching and mentoring a student, in addition to managing care for individual children. This afternoon's Well Teddy Clinic was hard work, but extremely interesting and satisfying – I really feel that I have had not just an influence on the health and well-being of individuals but also wider communities.

Jayne Price

Components of public health

Blair (2001) argued that every clinical encounter with patients should be inter-preted as an opportunity for health promotion and preventative care even in acute paediatric settings. An example of the sorts of ways a health visitor can influence child public health is described in Box 6.2. Children's nurses should be thinking the same way.

Box 6.2   A morning in the life of a health visitor

It is 9 a.m., as I sort through post, the telephone rings. It is Mrs Smith; she tells me that she hasn't slept for several nights since starting our sleep management pro-gramme for her 3-year-old son Josh. We talk through what she has done and I praise her for management and adherence to the programme we devised together. I reas-sure her that although things often get worse before they improve, that she should notice a difference by the end of the week. I encourage her in her motivation to con-tinue with the programme by pointing out the long-term benefits that success will make to her son's schooling and how her own mood will improve. I arrange to con-tact her again the following day to further evaluate her situation and offer ongo-ing support. As I document our contact, I reflect on how a parenting support group would be able to give Mrs Smith additional peer support; however, there is currently no group in the area.

The receptionist telephones and tells me that Mr Jones has arrived with his daugh-ter Jemma who is 18 months old. The family were concerned regarding their child's language development which is not as advanced as their neighbour's child of the same age. I complete a review of Jemma's progress and find that she is reaching developmental norms. I reassure her parent and discuss the importance of reading to Jemma and engaging her in conversation. There are a range of mother and toddler groups in the area. I suggest that Jemma's grandmother, who looks after her during the day; could take Jemma to one of these groups to encourage the child's interaction with her peers. On further discussion, I realise that the family have not taken Jemma for her MMR vaccine. Through questioning, I learn that there have been two con-straints: first, uncertainty regarding the safety of the vaccine and second, parental job insecurity has meant that the parents have felt unable to request time to take Jemma to the surgery's regular 2 p.m. session. The father has taken annual leave to attend today. Having discussed through concerns regarding the immunisation, obtained parental consent and a GP prescription, I arrange for Jemma to receive her Measles Mumps and Rubella (MMR) today.

It is now 10.15 a.m.; I leave the health centre for my first home visit of the day, in a deprived housing estate. I park my car as close as possible to the Green family's house; however, I still have to walk through dark and narrow passage ways, past boarded-up houses to reach the house. Mr Green greets me at the door. After a brief introduction and discussion of my role, I commence a family assessment and I com-plete an infant physical examination. Mr Green tells me that he has been smoking since he was 15 years old, he has tried to stop smoking twice before and failed. Now he does not know how he can successfully stop. He tells me that he really wants to stop smoking as he does not want to harm his baby and wants to be a long-lived, healthy and fit father. I commend his decision and discuss various smoking cessa-tion strategies and resources within the local area. Mr Green decides that he will use nicotine replacement therapy and join a local Healthy Living Centre 'stop smoking group'. I offer information on accessing these resources and arrange to contact him within a few days (to support his progress). The parents have not purchased a car safety seat; we discuss the legal and health implications of this. Mr Green lost his job just before the baby was born and financially things have been tight. The Trust has been running a safety scheme through which parents in hardship can buy safety equipment at reduced prices. After gaining the parent's permission, I will approach the scheme co-ordinator regarding the family's eligibility.

As I leave the house, I detour to the local community group and ask to speak to Jenny Gray, the community development officer. I ask whether there has been any response regarding our letter to the council housing environment in the estate. A council representative has agreed to arrange a meeting with the local residents, and I have been asked to attend. I suggest that Jenny contacts an environmental health officer who has also expressed concern regarding the deteriorating conditions in the estate and that I will speak to the health centre staff regarding a wider attendance. I return to my office in the health centre and speak to the Practice manager about the estate's local residence group.

It is now 12.30 and I have some time to further work on a local community 'health needs profile'. I find that in comparison with neighbouring locality rates, there is a lower incidence and duration of breastfeeding and higher obesity and postnatal depression rates. Many parents report difficulties in coping with their children's behaviours. I make an appointment with my line manager to discuss these health needs, so that we can initiate the development or commission services to meet local needs.

I stop for lunch and reflect on the different forms of family and community orientated public health activities that I have already engaged in today.

Janice Christie

The following section gives an overview of the principles involved in taking a public health perspective and provides a global overview as well as some specific examples.

The role of epidemiology in public health

Epidemiology is an important discipline in public health and is concerned the study of disease patterns in populations. 'Modern' interpretations of public health have also been influenced by the important contribution made by sociology (understanding the impact of socio-economic factors and ethnicity), geography (the impact of location) and political sciences (the growing impact of policy and involvement of population in decision making and inequality). It is not possible to review the role of all these disciplines in relation to public health; hence, particular reference is made to epidemiology.

Epidemiologists assess need usually by measuring disease frequency – the incidence and prevalence and through the compilation of routine statistics of death and disease (mortality and morbidity indicators). They also measure the burden of disease in populations using statistics on morbidity generated from various sources including routine information systems found in hospitals, general practices and child health surveillance systems. Although these information systems are vital for capturing information about births, immunisations, school health appointments, general practice registrations and information on deaths, there are a number of shortcomings that have been found mainly due to differences in recording and reporting practices. A good example is in relation to capturing information on children with developmental disorders (e.g. cerebral palsy, learning disability and autistic spectrum disorder). The problems in maintaining up-to-date information include problems around making a reliable diagnosis in these sorts of conditions, lack of standardised approaches in describing and classifying children by severity of the condition and lack of access for professionals to directly entering data into the information systems during clinical consultations. An example of how children's nurses can influence child public health through epidemiological work is described in Box 6.3.

Box 6.3   A day in the life of a nurse researcher

I am involved in a long-term project about children with cerebral palsy (CP). CP is a disorder of movement and posture caused by damage to the developing brain and a leading cause of significant physical disability in childhood. As an undergraduate nurse at Manchester University, I always really enjoyed and was interested in epidemiology – the science and study of disease patterns in populations, and I remembered choosing to study trends in perinatal morbidity and mortality as part of my epidemiology coursework. My day-to-day work involves running a dedicated, case register of children and young people with CP funded by the Department of Health, Social Security and Public Safety (Northern Ireland). The register is a confidential record of every child born with the condition or resident in the geographic region of Northern Ireland. My job involves the maintenance of the register: finding out about newly diagnosed children, capturing information about their clinical signs and symptoms including a brief birth history. I liaise closely with a paediatrician who validates that the children we think are potentially suitable for inclusion on the register have indeed got CP. The paediatrician does this by reviewing the data I have collated, which includes information on the distribution of abnormal tone and neurological signs and other information relating to medical diagnoses. Then I enter the data onto a statistical package on the computer, undertake checks on the data quality including accuracy of my data entry and then analyse and report on the number and changing trends in the condition over time. I report on this maybe once or twice a year to find out whether the condition is changing and in what ways. I do this work in collaboration with an epidemiologist who advises on statistical and registry methods and helps in the interpretation and writing up of the findings. Quite often, I am asked to come and present the findings to doctors, nurses, physiotherapists, parent support groups and voluntary agencies. Sometimes, parents ring me directly seeking more information about CP, or about the register and how to get involved.

The register is essentially a surveillance system which monitors the health of the childhood population in Northern Ireland in relation to this condition. There are four other similar registers of CP in the UK and around 16 across Europe. About once a year, all the registry teams meet up, to pool their data and explore trends and patterns in the epidemiology of CP across large populations as well as form collaborations to pursue additional research projects or analyses.

Although running and reporting on the register takes up about 3 days a week of my time, the remainder of my work focuses on developing research proposals often in collaboration with other researchers, professionals and parents; writing scientific papers and supervising nursing students undertaking higher degrees usually about children or young people with CP. A very important part of my work involves meeting and talking to families and to people with CP to help ensure the research takes account of their views but also their priorities for care, support and quality of life. Sometimes, I think that I would be more useful to families if I went back to work on a ward or in the community. Then I remember that my work along with many others in the field helps to keep the health and well-being of people with CP on the public health agenda.

Jackie Parkes

Public health interventions and their evidence

This area alone is potentially a huge topic, and there is no scope in this chapter to provide a comprehensive overview. Clinically effective interventions have three characteristics: they are based on the best evidence available, they achieve the intentioned health outcomes and care processes based on client's needs and they are subject to monitoring and review (CPHVA 1999). Often there is limited evidence available for many prevention-orientated public health nursing interventions.

The European Health 21 target 9 is that 'By the year 2020, there should be a significant and sustainable decrease in injuries, disability and death arising from accidents and violence in the Region' (WHO 1998). Accidents are the leading cause of male death, childhood death in 5–15 year olds and second highest reason for mortality in girls (Babb *et al*. 2002). Rates of accidental injury are highest among children from disadvantaged households (Drever and Whitehead 1997). Accidents can happen to children at home, school, childcare or while undertaking a journey. Different approaches to reduce childhood accidents have been reviewed systematically in the literature; most reviewers have indicated that there is a paucity of good evidence regarding various safety interventions.

There is little clear evidence that one-to-one advice provided by a health professional has an impact on the incidence of childhood injuries (Woods 2006), and the author suggested that enthusiastic professionals might make a more positive effect through campaigning for legislation and engineering change. The evidence for collective approaches to safety promotion such as legislative, community-based programmes and changes to the physical environment, however, is also limited. A recent systematic review (Ehiri *et al*. 2006) evaluated five studies regarding the effectiveness of interventions to increase the use of care booster seats for 5–7-year-old children. No evidence was found that booster seat laws increased usage (limited to one study that met the inclusion criteria); however, the authors commented that non-included studies that did not have a control (comparison) group suggested that legislation might have a positive effect. The provision of free booster seats, incentives and education were associated with more utilisation of the seats.

Given this limited evidence, how does the children's nurse tackle the issue of childhood safety? A first step is to keep well informed and up to date with growing evidence regarding childhood accidents and accident prevention and ensuring that this knowledge is transformed into everyday practice. Nurses can become actively involved with local or national bodies that promote childhood safety such as Royal Society for the Prevention of Accidents (RoSPA) and the Child Accident Prevention Trust or community development programmes. It is also possible to campaign for safety changes through professional bodies or local or national politicians. A further mechanism is to help move the frontiers of knowledge by undertaking research.

Collaborative working and public health

Recent international and national policy documents (WHO 1998, DH 1999b, 2004, Department of Health Social Services and Public Safety 2002) aim to improve in the health and well-being of adults and children through collaboration between different professional group and agencies. Collaborative working is also a fundamental principle of professional work undertaken to safeguard children (DH 1996, DHSSPSCNAC 1998). According to the Children NI Order (Department of Health and Social Services 1995) and Children Act (DH 1989), the welfare of the child is paramount in court proceedings, this means that children should be kept informed about what happens to them and that they should be encouraged to participate in decisions about their well-being. The law also requires that services should be provided in partnership with parents. The children's nurse has a responsibility to work collaboratively with other professionals by sharing concerns regarding the welfare of 'children in need' with other appropriate professionals such as social workers, family doctor, paediatrician, family health visitor or school nurse. Although current guidance and best practice regarding child health surveillance (Hall and Elliman 2003) and health promotion (Whitehead 2004) emphasises partnership and working with clients, there is some evidence that this may not always occur leaving some parents feeling excluded and others judged (Roche *et al.* 2005).

The Jakarta declaration (WHO 1997) stated the need to consolidate partnerships to improve health. The UK governmental policy has also championed the need for blurring professional boundaries and multi-agency working (DH 1999b, 2004, Department of Health Social Services and Public Safety 2002) and the importance of collaborative ways of working for nurses (Department of Health and Social Services 1998, DH 2002). Working together is also a key feature of 'Every child matters' (Department for Education and Skills 2003). Therefore, partnership working is an essential component of all child and health promotion interventions. Although there is recognition of the importance of inter-agency collaboration and provision of seamless services for users and carers, there is little evidence regarding what constitutes effective partnerships in health care. A literature review (Brown *et al.* 2006) of best business practices identifies that effective collaboration can be promoted by ensuring a positive vision for collaboration, ensuring that everyone involved has a stake in the success of the venture and ensuring that the right people are involved, relationships between people are managed so that factors enhancing trust, respect and participation are maximised and good communication is fostered. These are principles that children's nurses can adopt to promote better working practices in health care. Children's nurses also have a mandate to become involved with local commissioning of health services.

Conclusions and future developments

Public health essentially relates to collective or population well-being. Modern thought extends the definition to holistic health and equity. Such ideals are wholly compatible with Nursing & Medical Council (NMC) guidance and relevant to all practitioners of nursing. Ultimately, the future of public health and nursing will depend on how the ideas we have discussed in this chapter are facilitated within practice. Successful nursing public health activity depends on a dynamic partnership among research, education, management and the practitioner. Public health is dependent on working together with other professionals, agencies and local people to improve health and well-being of everyone. Given the warnings that health services will not be able to cope with future demand unless action is taken now to improve the well-being of the nation (Wanless 2002), it is imperative that children's nurses rise to the challenge and incorporate aspects of public health into everyday practice.

References

Babb P, Bird C, Bradford B, Burtenshaw S, Gardener D, Howell S, McConnell H, Myers K, Shipsey C and Upson A (2002). *Social Focus in Brief: Children*, London: National Statistics.

Bartlett JG and Hayden FG (2005). Editorial: Influenza A (H5N1): Will it be the next pandemic influenza? Are we ready? *Annals of Internal Medicine*, 143(6), 460–462.

Black D, Morris JN, Smith C and Townsend P (1980). *The Black Report*, London: Pelican Books.

Blair M (2001). The need for and the role of a coordinator in child health surveillance/promotion. *Archives of Disease in Childhood*, 84, 1–5.

Blair M, Stewart-Brown S, Waterson T and Crowther R (2003). *Child Public Health*. Oxford: Oxford University Press.

Brocklehurst N (2004). Public health and its implications for practice. *Nursing Standard*, 18(49), 48–54.

Brown D, White J and Leobbrandt L (2006). Collaborative partnerships for nursing faculties and health service providers: what can nursing learn from business literature? *Journal of Nursing Management*, 14, 170–179.

Butler J (1989). *Child Health Surveillance in Primary care: A Critical Review*. London: Her Majesty's Stationery Office.

Caplan G (1961). *An approach to Community Mental Health*. London: Tavistock Publications.

Council for the Education and Training of Health Visitors (1977). *An Investigation into the Principles of Health Visiting*. London: CETHV.

CPHVA (1999). *Clinical Effectiveness Information Pack*. London: CPHVA.

Craig P (2000). Nursing contribution to public health. In: Craig P and Lindsay GM (eds), *Nursing for Public Health. Population-Based Care*, Chapter 1, pp. 1–12. London: Churchill Livingstone.

Department for Education and Skills (2003). *Every Child Matters*. London: DFES.

Department of Health (DH) (1988). *Public Health in England: The Report of the Committee of Inquiry into the Future Development of the Public Health Function* (Acheson Report). London: HMSO.

Department of Health (DH) (1989). *The Children Act*. London: HMSO.

Department of Health (DH) (1996). *Childhood Matters. Report of the National Commission of Inquiry into the prevention of child abuse*. London: The Stationery Office.

Department of Health (DH) (1998). *Independent Inquiry into Inequalities in Health Report*, Sir Donald Acheson, C. (ed). London: The Stationery Office.

Department of Health (DH) (1999a). *Making a Difference: Strengthening the Nursing, Midwifery and Health Visiting Contribution to Health and Health Care*. London: DH.

Department of Health (DH) (1999b). *Saving Lives Our Healthier Nation*. London: Stationery Office.

Department of Health (DH) (2001). *Health Visitor Practice Development Pack*. London: DH publications.

Department of Health (DH) (2002). *Liberating the Talents*. London: HMSO.

Department of Health (DH) (2004). *Choosing Health, Making Healthier Choices Easier*. London: DH.

Department of Health (DH) (2007). Public Health in England (Archive CMO Feature-Last updated: 24/06/03) http://www.dh.gov.uk/en/Aboutus/.

Department of Health and Social Services (1995). *The Children's (NI) Order*. Belfast: HMSO, MinistersandDepartmentLeaders/ChiefMedicalOfficer/Features/FeaturesArchive/Browsable/DH_4102835, Department of Health, London (last accessed 1 March 2008).

Department of Health and Social Services (1998). *Valuing Diversity a Way Forward, a Strategy for Nursing, Midwifery and Health Visiting*. Belfast: DHSS.

Department of Health Social Services and Public Safety (2002). *Investing for Health*. Belfast: Department of Health Social Services and Public Safety.

Department of Health and Social Services Central Nursing Advisory Committee (DHSSPSCNAC) (1998). *Guidance on Professional Practice for Nurses, Midwives and Health Visitors. The Children (NI) Order 1995*. Belfast: DHSSPSCNAC.

Dinkevich E, Hupert J, and Moyer VA (2001). Evidence based well child care. *British Medical Journal*, 323(7317), 846–849.

Drever F and Whitehead M (1997). *Inequalities in Health, Decennial Supplement*. London: Office for National Statistics, The Stationery Office.

Ehiri JE, Ejere HOD, Magnussen L, Emusu D, King W and Osberg JS (2006). Interventions for promoting booster seat use in four to eight year olds travelling in motor vehicles. *The Cochrane Database of Systematic Reviews*, 4.

Faculty of Public Health (2008). What is public health http://www.fphm.org.uk/about_faculty/what_public_health/default.asp, Faculty of Public Health, London (accessed 10 February 2008).

Hall DM (1989). *Health for all Children*. Oxford: Oxford University Press.

Hall DMB (1999). School nursing: past, present and future. *Archives of Diseases in Childhood*, 81, 181–184.

Hall DMB and Elliman D (2003). *Health for all Children*. Oxford: Oxford University Press.

Hayes L (2005). Public health and nurses … what is your role? *Primary Health Care*. 15(5), 22–25.

Holman J (1992). Something old, something new: perspectives on five 'new' public health movements. *Health Promotion Journal of Australia*, 2(3), 4–11.

Hughes J and Horsburgh J (2002). The role of the community children's nurse: the perspective of a practitioner and an educator. *Current Paediatrics*, 12, 425–430.

Kuh D, Ben-Shlomo Y (eds) (1997). *A Life Course Approach to Chronic Disease Epidemiology: Tracing the Origins of Ill-Health from Early to Adult Life*. Oxford: Oxford Medical Publications.

Ledwith M (2005). *Community Development*. University of Bristol: The policy press.

Ministerial Group on the Family (1998). *Supporting Families, a consultation document*. London: The Stationery Office.

Naidoo J and Wills J (1994). *Health Promotion Foundations for Practice*. London: Balliere Tindall.

Nursing and Midwifery Council (NMC) (2004). *NMC Code of Professional Conduct. standards for conduct, performance and ethics*. London: NMC.

Office of National Statistics (ONS) (2002). *Children in the UK*. Press Release. ONS, London. Available from http://www.statistics.gov.uk/pdfdir/child0702.pdf.

Pomerleau J and McKee M (2005). The emergence of public health and the centrality of values. In: Pomerleau J and McKee M (eds), *Issues in Public Health. Understanding Public Health*, Chapter 1, pp. 5–7. England: Open University Press.

Porter D (1999). *Health, Civilization, and the State: A History of Public Health from Ancient to Modern Times*. London: Routledge.

Poulton B, Mason C, McKenna H, Lynch C and Keeney S (2000). *The Contribution of Nurses, Midwives and Health Visitors to the Public Health Agenda*. Belfast: Department of Health, Social Services and Public Safety.

Robinson J and Elkan R (1996). *Health Needs Assessment, Theory and Practice*. New York: Churchill Livingstone.

Roche B, Cowley S, Salt N, Scammell A, Malone M, Savile P, Aikens D and Fitzpatrick S (2005). Reassurance or judgement? Parents' views on the delivery of child health surveillance programmes. *Family Practice*, 22, 507–512.

Rosen G (1993). *A history of Public Health*. Baltimore: John Hopkins Press.

Ross A (2003). Promoting Health – Challenges for Children's Nurses. *Paediatric Nursing*, 15(4), 37–39.

Scottish Executive Health Department (2001). *Nursing for Health: A Review of the Contribution of Nurses, Midwives and Health Visitors to Improving the Public's Health in Scotland*. Edinburgh: SEHD.

Scottish Executive Health Department (2006). *The WHO Europe Family Health Nursing Pilot in Scotland. Final Report*. Edinburgh: SEHD.

Smith MA (2004). Health visiting: the public health role. *Journal of Advanced Nursing*, 45(1), 17–25.

Stewart-Brown J (2002). Research in Relation to Equity: Extending the Agenda. *Pediatrics*, 11(3), 763–765.

Tones K and Green J (2004). *Health Promotion*. London: Sage.

United Nations (1989). *Convention on the rights of the child* Treaty Series, Vol. 1577, United Nations, New York.

Wanless D (2002). Securing our health: Taking a long term view. In *Final report* Health Trends Team at HM Treasury, London.

Warren MD (2000). A Chronology of state medicine, public health welfare and related services in Britain 1066-1999 (http://www.fphm.org.uk/resources/AtoZ/r_chronology_of_state_medicine.pdf) The Faculty of public health medicine, London (last accessed 10 February 2008).

Whitehead D (2004). Health promotion and health education: Advancing the concepts. *Journal of Advanced Nursing*, 47(3), 311–320.

Wilson ME (1995). Travel and the emergence of infectious disease. *Emergent Infectious Disease*, 1(2), 39–46.

Woods A (2006). The role of health professionals in childhood injury prevention: A systematic review of the literature. *Patient Education and Counselling*, 64, 35–42.

World Health Organisation (WHO) (1978). *Declaration of Alma-Ata International Conference on Primary Health Care*, Alma-Ata, USSR, 6–12 September, WHO, Geneva.

World Health Organisation (WHO) (1986). *Ottawa Charter for Health Promotion*, WHO, Geneva.

World Health Organisation (WHO) (1997). *Jakarta Declaration on Leading Health Promotion into the 21st Century*, WHO, Geneva.

World Health Organisation (WHO) (1998). *HEALTH21: The Health for all Policy Framework for the WHO European Region*, World Health Organization Regional Office for Europe, Copenhagen.

World Health Organisation (WHO) (2000). *The Family Health Nurse: Context, Conceptual Framework and Definitive Curriculum*, WHO, Denmark.

Chapter 7

The Children and Young People's Mental Health Practitioner

Barry Nixon

Introduction

This chapter focuses on the current developments in mental health nursing practice with children and young people (CYP). It describes the knowledge, skills, competencies and capabilities required of those mental health practitioners working
with CYP. It also provides information that is relevant to children's commissioners
and providers of child and adolescent mental health training and education, with
a developing framework to prepare future CYP mental health practitioners for safe
and accountable practice in a range of CYP mental health settings.

Addressing core competencies that have common currency across universal
child and adolescent mental health services (CAMHS), this chapter will also define
some of the additional competencies for professional groups working in specialist CAMHS in health, education and social services. It will differentiate between
working in universal or primary services and working in specialist CAMHS.
Distinctions will also be made between working with different age groups of CYP.

Background: Historical context

In relation to many other branches of health care, child and adolescent mental
health is a very young specialism. The early child guidance movement established in the USA in the 1920s led to the development in the UK by 1939. With
the advent of the National Health Services (NHS) in 1948, most areas had a
rudimentary child guidance service, and by the 1970s, most boroughs and coun-
ties had at least out-patient services. In parallel with this development, although
running slightly behind it, separate development took place of mental health
departments for children and adolescents in NHS teaching hospitals. These
developments up to the mid-1970s were due in large part to advocacy by dedicated people rather than as a result of deliberate policy initiatives.

Between the mid-1970s and 1990, a number of policy changes influenced, both directly and indirectly, the development of CAMHS. Notable among these were the shift from basing policy on the needs of known service users to wider populations not necessarily known to services, the creation of area health authorities that took over much of the responsibility for public health from local authorities, including school medical services and staff employed in child guidance, whereas the employment of social workers in health passed in the opposite direction, from the NHS to the newly created social services departments. In addition, changes in the roles of social workers (primarily to address an increasing child protection agenda) and educational psychologists (to meet the increasing demand for statement of special educational needs) led to a rise in the importance of nurses and clinical psychologists within CAMHS.

It is arguable that the generally laudable and ground-breaking changes of 1974 unwittingly presaged the decline of the child guidance model of service delivery, left a vacuum in service models that was not filled until recently by the tiered strategic approach to service design. The publication of the thematic review by the NHS Health Advisory Service (HAS) in 1995 (Williams and Richardson 1995) provided a national thrust towards coherent service planning and commissioning of CAMHS. The review reported that CAMHS in England and Wales were very patchy. Despite the obvious energy and commitment of the staff, there were problems with the availability and accessibility of service, limited standardisation and replication of their work, and the priority of young people in need varied greatly across services in adjacent areas.

In recent years, the government has been striving to bring greater coherence to mental health services for CYP and to remove the inequalities in service provision highlighted by the Audit Commission. In 1999, the Department of Health announced new investment in CAMHS and issued a circular setting out how funds were to be used. In September 2002, improvement, expansion and reform (which set out the NHS priorities for the 2003–2006 planning round) set the expectation that comprehensive mental health services for CYP would be available in all areas by 2006; it also states that CAMHS is to be increased by at least 10% every year (in staffing, patient contacts and/or investment) according to local agreed priorities. In September 2004, the Children's National Service Framework (NSF) included the mental health and psychological well-being of CYP as one of its 11 standards.

Child and adolescent mental health

Mental health needs and problems of CYP are defined differently. Although all CYP have mental health needs, as many as one in five have mental health problems (Mental health foundation 1999) and as many as 1 in 10 aged 5–15 have a diagnosable mental health disorder (Green 2005).

Everyone has a role to play in ensuring that the mental health needs of CYP are met. In adopting this broad concept, there is the explicit acknowledgment that supporting CYP with mental health problems is *Everyone's Business*. Government policy and subsequent service development are increasingly aware that there is good reason to invest early to save later. Untreated mental health problems are linked to educational failure, family and social problems, crime and antisocial behaviour. Many unresolved mental health problems occurring in childhood continue into adulthood.

Mental health problems and disorders in CYP manifest in many ways; they can present in the way they feel, think and behave. The terms mental health problems and mental health difficulties should be clarified. Definitions range from the highly categorised employed by some health service professionals to those based on more descriptive terms that are prevalent in school environments. Although mental health problems can and often do interfere with a child's development and functioning, they are differentiated from mental disorders as being mild and transitory in nature to the child and the family. When a problem is particularly severe or persistent over time, or when a number of these difficulties are experienced at the same time, CYP are often described as having mental health disorders. The challenge for the child and adolescent mental health practitioner is to find ways in which the different approaches and frameworks and professionals can operate effectively together.

All professionals working with CYP have a responsibility to ensure that the CYP they work with are given every opportunity possible to reach their full potential and experience good mental health. Good mental health is commonly defined as having the ability to:

- Develop psychologically, emotionally, intellectually and spiritually.
- Initiate, develop and sustain mutually satisfying personal relationships.
- Use and enjoy solitude.
- Become aware of others and empathise with them.
- Play and learn.
- Develop a sense of right and wrong and.
- Resolve (face) problems and setbacks and learn from them.

Good mental health is also about emotional resilience. Resilience seems to involve several related elements. First, a sense of self-esteem and confidence, second a belief in one's own self-efficacy and ability to deal with change and adaptation and third, a repertoire of social problem solving approaches.

There is now rapidly expanding development of strategies to promote, prevent and intervene early to offset the possible development of mental health problems and disorders in CYP. All professionals working with CYP have a responsibility for promoting good mental health and prevent mental health problems and disorders. Primary mental health prevention refers to interventions aimed at the general population and focus on strategies to reduce the possibility of mental health problems occurring in the first place. Early intervention is intended to prevent mental health problems developing into mental health disorders. Mental health professions must endeavour to integrate these approaches into their work with CYP.

Defining CAMHS

Services that contribute towards the mental health and psychological well-being of CYP are provided by many agencies. CAMHS is a multi-agency activity, and nursing CYP with mental health problems takes place in an interagency context. The term CAMHS is a broad concept embracing all services that contribute to the mental health care of CYP, whether provided by health, education, social services, the youth justice system or other agencies. CAMHS cover all types of provision and intervention from mental health promotion and primary prevention through to very specialist care as provided by in-patient units for young people with mental illness. Interventions may be indirect for example consultative advice to another agency or direct therapeutic work with an individual child or family.

The NHS HAS report entitled 'Together We Stand' (HAS 1995) was the first national review of CAMHS. The review revealed wide variations across the country in relation to staffing and practices. However, the primary impact of the HAS report came from its recommendation to introduce a four-tier structure for CAMHS (see Fig. 7.1). This model remains the foundation, albeit with some local variations, for CAMHS in England, although the recent document *Every Child Matters* (Department for Education and Skills 2003) advocates a revised conceptualisation of CAMHS around more local integrated services such as children's

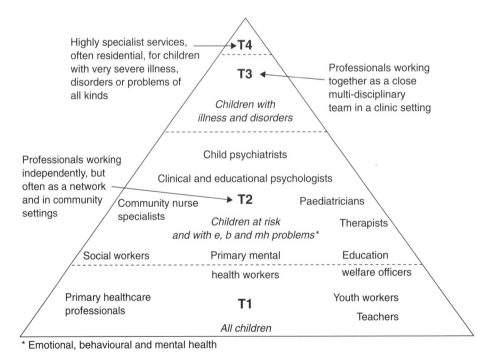

* Emotional, behavioural and mental health

Fig. 7.1 The four-tier structure of CAMHS.

trusts, focussing on five global outcomes – being healthy, staying safe, enjoying and achieving, making a positive contribution and achieving economic well-being.

The four-tier structure of CAMHS

CAMHS are provided in line with a four-tier strategic framework which is now widely accepted as the basis for planning, commissioning and delivering services (Table 7.1). The NHS HAS (1995) promulgated this model to produce a strategic

Table 7.1   Four-tier strategic framework.

Tier 1	The frontline of service delivery that is all professionals who have day-to-day contact with CYP; this includes general practitioners (GPs), health visitors, school nurses, teachers, social workers, youth justice workers, voluntary agencies and many more.
	Practitioners at this level will be able to offer general advice and treatment for less severe problems, contribute towards mental health promotion, identify problems early in their development, and refer to more specialist services.
Tier 2	Provided by specialist-trained mental health professionals, this can include primary mental health workers, psychologists and counsellors working in GP practices, paediatric clinics, schools and youth services. Practitioners at this level tend to be CAMHS specialists working in community and primary care settings in a uni-disciplinary way. Practitioners offer consultation to families and other practitioners, outreach to identify severe or complex needs that require more specialist interventions, assessment which may lead to treatment at Tiers 3 or 4 and training to practitioners at Tier 1.
Tier 3	Usually a multi-disciplinary team or service working in a community mental health clinic or child psychiatry outpatient service, providing a specialised service for CYP with more severe, complex and persistent disorders. Team members are likely to include child and adolescent psychiatrists, social workers, clinical psychologists, community psychiatric nurses, child psychotherapists, occupational therapists and family, art, music and drama therapists. May be offered as a 'hub and spoke' model with Tier 2 and some Tier 3 functions delivered locally, and more specialised Tier 3 activities provided at central but accessible locations.
Tier 4	Very specialised services in residential, day patient or out-patient settings for children and adolescents with severe and/or complex problems requiring a combination or intensity of interventions. Can include secure forensic adolescent units, eating disorders units, specialist neuro-psychiatric teams, and other specialist teams. Tier 4 provision also includes day care and residential facilities provided by sectors other than the NHS, such as residential schools, and very specialised residential social care settings including specialised therapeutic foster care. It is common for Tier 4 services to be commissioned on a sub-regional, regional or supra-regional basis.

approach with the intention to integrate the many elements of a truly comprehensive service for children, adolescents and young people into an understand-
able whole. The model is further re-stated and redefined in the NSF (Department
for Education and Skills and Department of Health 2004). The model intended,
through encouragement of the development of service networks, to support
those working with children, young people and families, so that they are enabled
in their work and their skills are increased, with a view to reducing the consequence of staff from specialist services being overwhelmed by referral of problems that may be more helpfully addressed in the community by other service
components.

Although there is some variation in the way the framework has been developed
and applied across the country, the tiered concept has provided a language that
has bridged different sectors of care and different professions and enabled focused
discourse around which services should be provided for whom and by whom.
There are differing interpretations of the tiered strategic approach. Arguably, these
differences are less important than achieving clarity about the functions required
of services and the effective commissioning of comprehensive CAMHS that are
tailored to the needs of children, young people and families locally.

Interpretation of the four-tier model

The four-tier strategic concept is now accepted as policy in both England and
Wales. It is widely recognised that the majority of CYP with mental health problems will be seen at Tiers 1 and 2. However, it is increasingly recognised that
neither CYP nor services meeting local need fit neatly into a structural interpretation of the tiers. CYP's journeys involve movement through services as their
condition is recognised as more complex or as and when conditions are amel-
iorated. Some children need to utilise a number of services that can involve and
span each or all of the CAMHS tiers at the same time.

The four-tier model is not so much a structural approach to service delivery
as a design tool. The model is not intended as a template that must be applied
rigidly but rather as a conceptual framework for ensuring that a comprehensive
range of services is commissioned and available to meet all the mental health
needs of CYP in an area, with clear referral routes between tiers.

Since the HAS report was published in 1995, numerous policy documents
have followed including Quality Protects (Department of Health 1998), The
Crime and Disorder Act (1998) and The NHS Plan (Department of Health 2000).
The NSF (Department of Health 2004) set new standards and defined future
service models for children across NHS and social care settings and has had
an impact on the contexts in which professionals who work with CYP practice.
The needs of children, young people and their families are now at the centre of
all the mental health practitioner does in organising, planning and delivering
mental health and other children's service (McDougall 2004). The NSF is underpinned by an implementation strategy designed to provide support for parents

and carers, early intervention and effective protection, accountability, integration and workforce reform. The NSF is part of a wider developmental strategy referred to as the Change for Children Programme.

The current workforce

More than 4 million people in England work with CYP or support those working with CYP (Department for Education and Skills and Department of Health 2004). This includes 2.4 million paid staff and 1.8 million unpaid staff and volunteers. Nurses continue to be the single largest professional group in specialist CAMHS, making up ~26% of the current workforce (CAMHS Mapping 2005) Those nurses in Tier 1 CAMHS will come from various professional backgrounds and are currently practising as children's nurses, school nurses, registered general nurses and health visitors. Several groups of nurses are working as autonomous practitioners in specialist CAMHS at Tiers 2, 3 and 4 (Leighton *et al.* 2001). Although most are mental health nurses, increasing numbers of children's nurses are entering the speciality as well as smaller numbers of learning disability nurses (Jones 2003). An increasing number of nurses are also primary mental health workers, practising at the interface between Tier 1, initial contact services and specialist CAMHS (Gale *et al.* 2005).

What is clear is that the CYP service workforce is diverse, with people entering at various stages in their lives, and includes workers who will have little or no specific training for working with children who have mental health problems. Many primary level practitioners to feel discomfort with engaging with young people with mental health problems, 'developing and expanding the expertise of primary care and community practitioners in child and adolescent mental health offers an opportunity to improve access to services that are acceptable to their children and their families, leaving specialists free to work with children and families have complex and severe needs' (Macdonald and Bower 2000).

The needs of CYP are different from those of adults, and those working in this area will require particular skills, knowledge and competencies to meet these needs. Despite this, much education and training for key professionals continue to neglect child and adolescent mental health. Education and training programmes should have common currency for all those working with CYP and should prepare them with the knowledge, skills and attitudes to work in a range of multi-disciplinary and interagency settings. Current education and training programmes however do not necessarily provide the necessary knowledge, skills and competencies to understand, care for or treat CYP with mental health problems (McDougall 2004), and nursing branch programmes do not necessarily produce nurses who are fit for practice in CAMHS settings (Hooton 1999, RCN 2003). The lack of education and training has seen the development of several local and regional education and training programmes evolving. Many of these training programmes are being modelled on the newly developed capability frameworks and are currently being reviewed in the context of their fitness for purpose and impact on CAMHS delivery (DH 2007, National Workforce Programme 2007).

The importance for all professionals who work with CYP to have a basic understanding of child and adolescent mental health is now widely acknowledged and well documented (Welsh Assembly Government 2001, Department for Education and Skills 2003, Department of Health 2004, NHS Education for Scotland 2004). Few would disagree that all professionals who are responsible for the health, education and welfare of CYP should possess the knowledge, skills, competencies and capabilities needed to address their mental health needs. The need to improve the experience and outcomes for CYP has led to the development of various standards against which the quality of care being delivered and services themselves can be measured.

National occupational standards (NOS) for mental health and children are available, and social care services currently have various occupational standards relating to the care of CYP (Department for Education and Skills 2003). The purpose of the NOS for Mental Health is to help raise the standard of practice by providing a competence framework for each key role against which performance may be assessed and measured. Occupational standards can be used as a tool for workforce management and specification tasks such as appraisal, personal development planning and performance management.

The NHS Knowledge and Skills Framework (KSF) is to facilitate the development of services, so that they better meet the needs of service users, to help in the development and review of staff working in the NHS. As the NHS KSF is a broad generic framework that focuses on the application of knowledge and understanding, it does not describe the exact knowledge and understanding that people need to develop. The exact knowledge and understanding required for the delivery of mental health services comes from the NOS for Mental Health which then provides evidence towards the achievement of the appropriate dimension in the KSF.

The majority of frameworks are based on a common principle that there is a need for a universal and generic service for all CYP and that the complexity of level of service provided will increase as does the level of need of the child. The Sainsbury Centre report, 'The Capable Practitioner' (Sainsbury Centre for Mental Health and National Institute for Mental Health in England 2001), introduced the concept of an increasingly specialised level of service and used it to provide a framework and list of practitioner capabilities required to implement *The National Service Framework for Mental Health* (Department of Health 1999). The Capability Framework combines the notion of the reflective practitioner with that of the effective practitioner. This framework may be useful in looking at the competencies needed by the workforce across sectors, responsible for delivering the NSF for Children, Young People and Maternity Services and Change for Children Programme: Every Child Matters.

The Sainsbury Centre (2001) suggested that a competency describes the level of expertise expected within a particular domain of capability.

In thinking about the development of core competencies in CAMHS, it is acknowledged that not all professionals need them at the same level. For example a Connexions worker will require basic understanding of mental health and knowledge of common mental health problems, whereas a more in depth understanding will be required by a specialist nurse, psychologist or psychiatrist. As nurses enter a particular speciality, it is likely that they will become more knowledgeable and proficient in that area. It is acknowledged that different levels of capability are appropriate between the different service providers. For example the knowledge that a school nurse may have of mental health problems and disorders will develop as their experience does. However, it would be inappropriate for them to develop it to a level of say a nurse specialist working in a Tier 3 CAMHS.

A capability framework

In 2001, the Children and Young People's Unit published 'Building a Strategy for Children and Young People' (Department for Education and Skills 2001). This set out proposed capabilities for those working with children, young people and their families or carers and is consistent with workforce recommendations in the NSF for Children, Young people and Maternity Services (Department of Health 2004), the Change for Children Programme, Every Child Matters (Department for Education and Skills 2003) and the youth green paper, 'Youth Matters' (Department for Education and Skills 2005).

CYPU – Strategy 2001 – Recommendations for services

- *Centred on the needs of the child or young person*: the best interests of the child or young person should be paramount, taking into account their wishes and feelings.
- *High quality*: policies and services should aspire to reach high standards of quality for the benefit of the CYP they serve.
- *Family orientated*: full recognition should be given to family members, including extended family members who contribute to the well-being of the child or young person.
- *Equitable and non-discriminatory*: all CYP should have access to services that they need, when they need them and in a way which respects diversity, equality and individuality.
- *Inclusive*: policies and services should be sensitive to the individual needs and aspirations of every child and young person, taking full account of their race, ethnicity, gender, sexual orientation, ability or disability.
- *Empowering*: CYP should be given the opportunity to play an effective role in the design and delivery of policies and services.
- *Results orientated and based on evidence*: high-quality research, evaluation, monitoring and review should ensure that decisions that effect CYP are well informed.
- *Coherent service design and delivery*: services should work together in a coherent, comprehensive and integrated way.
- *Supportive and respectful*: policies and services should be delivered in a manner that is respectful and supportive of CYP.
- *Community enhancing*: communities should be empowered to make positive changes for their CYP, so that improvements can be owned and sustained locally.

Children and young persons mental health practitioner and the 10 essential shared capabilities

The 10 Essential Shared Capabilities (ESC) describe the underpinning values and principles required to deliver appropriate and effective services for people with mental health problems. The purpose of the 10 ESC is to set out the shared or common capabilities that all staff working in mental health services should achieve as a minimum. These capabilities form the core building blocks for the education, learning, teaching and training of all staff working in CYP services whether they be professionally qualified or not and whether they work in the NHS, social care or in the statutory and private and voluntary sector:

1. Working in partnership.
2. Respecting diversity.
3. Practising ethically.
4. Challenging inequality.
5. Promoting recovery.
6. Identifying people's needs and strengths.
7. Providing child- and family-centred care.
8. Making a difference.
9. Promoting safety and positive risk taking.
10. Personal development and learning.

1. Working in partnership

Partnership working is part and parcel of modern practice. All those working with CYP, their families and carers should aim to develop and maintain constructive working relationships. It is becoming increasingly essential to be able to effectively work across a range of multi-disciplinary and interagency teams and networks. Various creative approaches are needed if we are to improve participation and user involvement and enhance partnership working in CYP services.

2. Respecting diversity

When working with CYP possessing the knowledge, skills and attitudes to respect diversity, provide choice and deliver child or young person–centred services are essential. This is to ensure that interventions are appropriate to the child or young person's age, race, culture, disability, gender, spirituality and sexuality. CYP, their families and carers can then enjoy ready access and make meaningful choices about the mental health care.

3. Practising ethically

To practice ethically and fulfil their professional obligations, those working with CYP must be able to recognise the rights and responsibilities of service users and their families and carers, acknowledging power differentials and minimise them whenever possible. It is essential that those working with CYP understand their professional duties in relation to confidentiality, consent and the rights of the people they work with in the context of providing mental health services for CYP. It is also important to have a good understanding of children's legislation, mental health law and know how to interpret the relevant provisions of these legal frameworks in their daily practice.

4. Challenging inequality

Helping to create, develop and maintain valued social roles for CYP and their families is essential to the mental health prevention agenda and an important part of social inclusion, recovery and normalisation for those who are already receiving mental health services. Historically, some particular groups of CYP have previously received a poor CAMHS such as minority ethnic groups (Mental Health Act Commission 2004), young people aged 16 and 17 and those with a learning disability or pervasive developmental disorder.

5. Promoting recovery

Working in partnership to provide care and treatment that enables CYP, their families and carers to tackle mental health problems with hope and optimism is essential. By assisting CYP, their families work towards a valued lifestyle within and beyond the limits of their mental health problems; they can be helped to enhance social functioning, inclusion and overall quality of life for CYP with mental health problems.

6. Identifying people's needs and strengths

The core business of CAMHS is to develop mental health and psychological well-being, prevent mental disorder and provide support when CYP suffer mental health problems and disorders. It is essential that those working with CYP can recognise and build on strengths and resilience factors in the child or young person, their family or carers.

7. Providing child- and family-centred services

Negotiating meaningful and achievable goals is fundamental to successful assessment and treatment and is essential from the perspective of CYP and their families. The mental health practitioner must be able to identify treatment outcomes for CYP, their families or carers.

8. Making a difference

Facilitating access to and delivering the best quality, evidence-based, value-based health and social care interventions to meet the needs and aspirations of service users and their families are central to the role of working child mental health services.

9. Promoting safety and positive risk taking

Depending on their age, maturity and the level of understanding, those working with CYP must ensure safety at all times while promoting therapeutic risk in an attempt to empower CYP, their families and carers. This includes working with the tension between promoting safety and positive risk taking.

10. Personal development and learning

The need to keep up to date with changes in practice and participating in life-long learning, taking part in personal and professional development for one's self through supervision, appraisal and reflective practice is essential for those working with CYP.

CYP's mental health practitioner: Common core skills, knowledge and competencies

Although the following capabilities are not exhaustive, the following range of skills, knowledge and competence can be described as essential for CYP mental health practitioner.

Core capabilities for all who work with children

Understanding mental health and psychological well-being

All professionals should be able to recognise and understand a wide range of different behaviours and know when to ask for assistance. As a minimum, the mental health practitioner should be supported to understand issues in relation to mental health, and psychological well-being should include opportunities to develop the awareness, knowledge, skills, attitudes and strategies in relation to.

Mental health promotion, illness prevention and early intervention

Those in contact with children need to be able to have sufficient knowledge of children's mental health to identify those who need help, offer advice and support to those with mild or minor problems and have sufficient knowledge of specialist services to be able to refer on appropriately when necessary (Department of Health 2004). The mental health practitioner should possess the knowledge, skills and attitudes relevant to mental health promotion, education, prevention and early intervention strategies for child and adolescent mental health (Department of Health 2004).

Communication

The mental health practitioner should have an understanding of appropriate communication strategies with CYP and their families, as well as carers, community members and other children's professionals. This should include skills for engaging, motivating, listening and reflecting during assessment and treatment with CYP. Communicating at a level that is appropriate to the child or young person's age, development and understanding requires a broad range of communication skills and strategies.

Understanding mental ill-health

The mental health practitioner should be able to assess the mental health needs of CYP and their families or carers. This should include the ability to recognise mental ill-health and mental health problems and disorders. Early identification of mental health problems in CYP is as follows:

- Factors and processes that can lead to mental ill-health.
- Diagnosis of mental illness and stigma as it relates to CYP.
- The various models of understanding mental health and illness (e.g. a medical perspective and a social perspective).
- Child and adolescent psychiatric disorders and skills to assess needs and identify appropriate ways to meet these needs.

Knowledge of current legislation and policy

Those working with CYP must keep up with the changing face of service provision, legislation and best practice as it affects CYP. The mental health practitioner should have knowledge of relevant legislation and the national policy context for multi-agency children's services and how it applies to their practice and organisation in which they work. They should understand and know how to use policies and procedures in relation to safeguarding children, consent to treatment, confidentiality and information sharing.

Knowledge about CYP services

It is important that those working with CYP have an understanding of the strategic context in which they work. The mental health practitioner should have knowledge of services provided to children by health, social services, education, youth justice and the voluntary sector.

Understanding the context and impact of socio-economic cultural, ethnic and gender issues

All those working with CYP should have an understanding of the context and impact of socio-economic, cultural, ethnic and gender issues on the mental health of children, adolescents and their families. The mental health practitioner will need an awareness of social inequalities and social exclusion and how these affect mental health and other developmental processes, differences in terms of access to resources and opportunities according to socio-economic status the ability to engaging CYP and their families from vulnerable groups.

Improving access to CAMHS

It is essential that all working with CYP have opportunities to develop the awareness, knowledge, skills, attitudes and strategies in relation to the identification, assessment, intervention and referral strategies for CYP, their families and carers and communities as it relates to mental health and emotional well-being.

Strategic problem solving and care planning

All those working with CYP should understand assessment frameworks and develop awareness of the law, code of professional conduct and other guidance applicable to information sharing. The mental health practitioner will be able to demonstrate knowledge and skills to anticipate and identify challenges to deliver CYP services and develop strategies for creative problem solving and local solutions.

Challenging inequality

All those working with CYP will need to be sensitive to the particular needs of CYP from minority ethnic groups. The mental health practitioner should be supported to develop the awareness, knowledge, skills, attitudes and strategies in relation to establishing and maintaining dialogue with regard to difference and diversity in terms of age, race, culture, disability, gender, spirituality and sexuality. They should also have the knowledge about differences and power inequalities between communities and groups who may be socially excluded and the impact on the mental health and psychological development of CYP.

Recovery and rehabilitation

Working in partnership with CYP, their families and carers is essential if those working with CYP are to promote recovery and rehabilitation and enhance social functioning and quality of life. To do this effectively, the mental health practitioner should be able to demonstrate knowledge and skills to enable CYP, their families and carers to manage transitions and access aftercare services, identify appropriate community-based support and aftercare systems, provide effective psycho-education and family support interventions.

Safety and positive risk taking

Those who work with CYP should focus on understanding protocols that promoting and safeguarding the welfare of CYP, knowing who to contact to express concerns, understanding protective factors and understanding how CYP manage risk themselves. The mental health practitioner should be able to demonstrate the knowledge and skills to safeguard and protect the safety and welfare of CYP, recognise, identify and assess risk factors and also to promote safe practise for themselves and others.

Continuing professional development

Keeping up to date with changes in practice and participating in lifelong learning involves personal and professional development for oneself and colleagues through supervision, appraisal and reflective practice. It is also an essential part of the children's clinical governance agenda. All those working with CYP should be able to demonstrate awareness, knowledge, skills and attitudes to reflect on practice and to identify strengths and weaknesses in own practice and evaluate personal and professional development needs in relation to the needs of child mental health service provision and the organisation within which they work.

Age-related core capabilities

Many of the skills required by those working with infants, pre-school or primary school children will be different from those needed by nurses who work with adolescents or young adults. Indeed, the Children's Commissioner in England, Al Aynsley-Green once famously suggested that there is no such thing as a child. By this, he meant that there are seven stages of childhood: the foetus, the neonate, the infant, the pre-school child, the school-age child, the adolescent and the transition to adulthood. To meet the mental health needs of children at different ages, nurses should have a good understanding of developmental theory and of physical, psychological and social developmental milestones. They should also understand the impact of trauma and adversity, abuse and other acute or chronic life stresses on the development and mediation of mental health and illness in children of different ages. There are a number of specific capabilities that those working with particular age groups should possess.

Working with expectant parents and infants

Pregnancy brings many emotional, physical and social changes for the mother, her partner and the rest of the family. The perinatal period, from conception until 2 years after childbirth, places the mother at heightened risk of mental health problems including postnatal depression (Royal College of Psychiatrists 2000). For those working with expectant parents and pre-school children, knowledge of pre-birth development and factors that impact on the perinatal period are of central importance.

Working with children aged between 0 and 4

For those who work with children during the early years, it is important to understand the needs of infants as well as the role of the parental relationship and the impact of this on the development of the child. The mental health practitioner will also need to understand the processes involved in parenting, the needs of parents and the impact of parenting on the development of the child. Support should be provided to the mental health practitioner, prepare them to meet the mental health needs of children during the early years and should address key aspects of attachment theory, the development of parent–child relationships and normal expected milestones in relation to physical, psychological and social functioning.

Working with primary school-aged children

For those working with CYP aged between 5 and 11, understanding of the role of the school and the family in the development of the child becomes increasingly important. It is also essential to understand the development, purpose and function of social and peer relationships and the beginning of independence and separation from the child's family or carers. In relation to children within their families, an understanding of the impact of siblings, sibling relationships, birth position, single parenthood and the different sorts of family and kinship structures is crucially important in understanding mental health risk and resilience factors. Life events affect children differently according to their age and the nature and degree of supportive and protective factors. Not only do separations, bereavements, disruption, abuse and trauma affect some children more than others, parents too vary in their abilities to contain, support and effectively manage their children as they grow up and approach adolescence.

Working with young people aged 12–18

During the adolescent period, the role of friends and the influence of the media becomes increasingly important. Those working with this age group should have knowledge of the 'the peer group' as a concept and its positive and negative influences on the young person's mental health and emotional resilience. They should also understand the nature of exploratory and risk-taking behaviours and be able to recognise and help develop factors and influences that may be protective during the teenage years.

Mental health practitioner in specialist CAMHS

The intention of this chapter is to focus on the education and training needs of those working across the range of services who currently work with CYP. In preparing the mental health practitioner to work in specialist CAMHS, additional competencies need to be developed to be able to assess and treat CYP with complex, severe or persistent mental health problems and disorders.

Mental health practitioner working in advanced, specialist or expert roles in CAMHS must possess advanced, specialist or expert practice knowledge, skills and competencies. Education and training should be provided by higher education institutions and academic centres and the role and profile of lecturer/ practitioners and link tutors should be maximised to support CAMHS nurses to link theory and practice. The mental health practitioner will be in key positions to receive and provide education and training from and to their CAMHS colleagues. The identification of core competencies for the specialist CAMHS workforce is currently being developed (Skills for Health 2007), by skills for health and specialist CAMHS.

Core competences for the specialist CAMHS workforce

The competencies identified for specialist CAMHS are currently being developed. These describe the functions appropriate to all individuals working in and delivering specialist CAMHS, in that they are generic. Individual practitioners will need to add competences related to their specific role and practice to produce a complete individual competence role profile. The current specialist core competencies include:

1. Communicate with CYP and those involved in their care.
2. Enable CYP to understand their health and well-being.
3. Recognise and respond to possible abuse of CYP.
4. Support CYP to cope with changes to their health and well-being.
5. Assess the effectiveness of individualised care plans in meeting the health and well-being needs of CYP.
6. Develop individualised care plans with CYP.
7. Work with CYP to assess their health and well-being.
8. Enable individuals and families to identify factors affecting, and options for optimising, their mental health and social well-being.
9. Implement interventions with CYP and those involved in their care.
10. Evaluate interventions with CYP and those involved in their care.
11. Take responsibility for the continuing professional development of self and others.
12. Support stakeholders in improving environments and practices to promote mental health.
13. Synthesise new knowledge into the development of your own practice.
14. Develop and sustain effective working relationships with staff in other agencies.
15. Promote the equality diversity rights and responsibilities of individuals.
16. Promote the values and principles underpinning best practice.
17. Involving young people in shaping service provision.

Conclusion and future challenges

Workforce issues remain the most significant challenge to the implementation of the changes and developments outlined in the NSF for Children and as identified in Every Child Matters, Children's Workforce Strategy.

A critical mass of staffing is required for services to be safe, timely and effective and able to respond to the wide range of needs that include specialist and multi-disciplinary services (Tiers 2, 3 and 4), support, consultation and face-to-face work within primary care settings (Tier 1), teaching, training, consultation and liaison, research and audit. Demographic factors including an ageing population, fewer school leavers and a healthy economy all indicate a need to be more imaginative in how we expand our workforce. It is now widely recognised and acknowledged that the development of a competent and capable children's workforce is a long-term strategy.

The enhanced role of the mental health practitioner in Tier 1 will assist in preventing mental health problems and ensuring prompt earlier intervention. They will require skills in child mental health, assistance with integrating new abilities into their roles in working with children and families and relationships and formalised support networks between them and professionals within specialist CAMHS.

The roles of specialist practitioners at Tier 2 are emerging. They include defined tasks (e.g. triage, assessment and intervention) performed by mental health practitioners working in community outpatient teams. These increasingly diverse activities will require experienced, autonomous practitioners. Other roles for mental health practitioners include those areas such as the Youth Offending Teams, work with looked after children, partnerships with social workers and fostering agencies, and work with young people who misuse substances. In many specialist CAMHS, the role of the primary mental health worker (PMHW) has been established. PMHWs are Tier 2 staff working at the interfaces between Tier 1 and specialist CAMHS. The role offers a range of enhanced practice opportunities in a unique way.

At Tier 3, the mental health practitioner will have the opportunity to develop as therapists and specialists providing input to programmes for specific mental health needs such as early onset psychosis, self-harm, eating disorders, autistic spectrum disorders and attention/deficit hyperactivity disorder (ADHD). This tier provides opportunities for mental health practitioners to become involved with developing multi-disciplinary resource centres that offer sessional and day care interventions to a range of CYP, assertive outreach teams and peripatetic forensic teams.

Future mental health practitioners will develop their expertise in inpatient settings, at Tier 4, especially with adolescents, and other very specialised commitments include those within inpatient forensic mental health teams.

The role of the mental health practitioner will continue to change and develop. There is a recognition that the capacity of the workforce must be developed and that the creation of new roles and workers will allow this to occur. This also requires the identification and availability of the necessary education and training to support this. Other future challenges will include new roles under mental health legislation, more changes in clinical practice, greater attention to health promotion and increasing service user autonomy.

The growing body of knowledge and skill and government commitments now provide profound opportunities for mental health practitioners to become involved in some of the most innovative programmes at all tiers of CAMHS. Future mental health practitioners are likely to have enormous influence in shaping new ways of helping children with mental health needs and contributing to developing comprehensive services built on an evolving evidence base.

Education and training for the children and young person's mental health practitioner must be consistent with wider children's workforce strategy and future education, and training should be commissioned and provided and evaluated in an interagency context. The future development of the child and adolescent mental health workforce is not only about skills and competencies but also about creating a shared understanding, shared vision and effective partnerships.

References

Audit Commission (1999). *Children in Mind: Child and Adolescent Mental Health Services.* Oxford: Audit Commission.

Department for Education and Skills (2005). *Youth Matters.* London: TSO.

Department for Education and Skills (DfES) and Department of Health (DH) (2004). National Service Framework for Children, Young People and Maternity Services: Children and Young People Who Are Ill. London: DH.

Department of Health (1998). Moving to Mainstream: The Report of a National Inspection of Services for Adults with Learning Disabilities. London: HMSO.

Department of Health (1999). *National Service Framework for Mental Health.* London: HMSO.

Department of Health (2000). Framework for the Assessment of Children in Need and Their Families. London: HMSO.

Department of Health (2004). *National Service Framework for Children, Young People and Maternity Services.* London: HMSO.

Department of Health (2005). *National Child and Adolescent Mental Health Service Mapping Exercise.* London: HMSO.

Department of Health (2007). A Learning and Development Toolkit for the Whole of the Mental Health Workforce across both Health and Social Care. London: DH.

Gale F, Hassett A and Sebuliba D (2005). *The Competency and Capability Framework for Primary Mental Health Workers in Child and Adolescent Mental Health Services* (CAMHS). London: National CAMHS Support Service.

Green (2005) In: McDougall T (2006). *Child and Adolescent Mental Health Nursing,* Blackwell.

Hooton S (1999). Who teaches nurses about child and adolescent mental health? *Paediatric Nursing,* 11(3), 10.

Jones N (2003). Training. In: *Child and Adolescent Mental Health Services: An Operational Handbook.* London: Gaskell.

Leighton S, Smith C, Minns K and Crawford P (2001). Specialist child and adolescent mental health nurses: A force to be reckoned with? *Mental Health Practice,* 5(2), 8–13.

Macdonald W and Bower P (2000) Child and adolescent mental health and primary care – current status and future directions. *Current Opinion in Psychiatry,* 13, 369–373.

McDougall T (2004). Listen and Learn. *Nursing Standard,* 19(6), 58.

Mental Health Act Commission (2004). Safeguarding Children and Adolescents Detained Under the Mental Health Act 1983 on Adult Psychiatric Wards. London: CSO Norwich.

Mental Health Foundation (1999). *Bright Futures.* London: Mental Health Foundation.

Mental Health Foundation (2002). *Turned Upside Down: Developing Community Based Crisis Services for 16–25 Year Olds Experiencing a Mental Health Crisis.* London: Mental Health Foundation.

NHS Education for Scotland (2004). *Promoting the Well-being and Meeting the Mental Health Needs of Children and Young People: A Development Framework for Communities, Agencies and Specialists Involved in Supporting Children, Young People and Their Families.* Edinburgh: NHS Education for Scotland.

NHS Health Advisory Service (1995). *Together We Stand: The Commissioning, Role and Management of Child and Adolescent Mental Health Services.* London: HMSO.

Royal College of Psychiatrists (2000). *Perinatal Maternal Mental Health Services. Council Report: CR88.* London: Royal College of Psychiatrists.

Sainsbury Centre for Mental Health and National Institute for Mental Health in England (NIMHE) (2001). *Essential Shared Capabilities*. London: SCMH.

Skills for health (2007). http://www.skillsforhealth.org.uk/page/ (accessed December 2007).

Welsh Assembly Government (2001). *Everybody's Business: Improving Mental Health in Wales – A CAMHS Strategy*. Cardiff: National Assembly for Wales.

Williams R and Richardson G (1995). *Together We Stand, the Commissioning, Role and Management of Child and Adolescent Mental Health Services*. London: HMSO.

Chapter 8
The Practitioner Working with Children and Young People with Disabilities

Jane Hughes, Gill Gibson and Joanna Assey

Introduction

This chapter will focus on the broad area of children with disabilities and the needs of both the children and their families. An overview of the historical development of this field of nursing will be given, followed by an introduction to the current situation. The later part of the chapter will then focus more specifically on the roles of practitioners working with children with disabilities and the skills and training needed to support children and their families. Examples from practitioners working with children and families with disabilities are also included.

History developments

The care and support of children and young people with disabilities has evolved significantly over recent years. This has reflected changes in both the society and the way in which health and social care services have been delivered.

An example of how care and support for children and young people has changed over the years is perhaps illustrated in the language used in referring to individuals with learning disabilities. Historically, terms such as subnormality, mental defective, imbecile, lunatic, idiot, feebleminded have been recorded. More recently, 'mental handicap' is a term used in the past 20 years and relates to a part on the nursing register. This was changed in the early 1990s to 'learning disabilities' (Northfield 2003).

People with learning disabilities have been separated from society and had many different labels attached to them as indicated previously, which it can be claimed have been given for scientific reasons to assist with diagnosis within a medical model of care. However, in today's culture, the use of such terms may appear derogatory. Thompson (2003) argues that attention to labels and language is a major plank in anti-discriminatory practice.

In recent years, the broader term of 'children with a disability' is used, and this can include children and young people with physical disabilities, learning disabilities, a sensory impairment or a combination of all which could be defined as complex needs or even life-threatening illnesses. Warner (2006) suggests that definition-based physiological assumptions do not serve children and their families well, as they do not reflect societal attitude and acceptance. Today, labels such as learning disabilities, intellectually disabled, mental retardation and 'challenging behaviour' are used to describe individuals' difficulties, and through discourse, the label takes on the personality and the individual may be lost. A case in point is a definition from the Children's Act 1989 and states that

> ... a child is disabled if 'he is blind, deaf or dumb, suffers from mental disorder of any kind or is substantially an permanently handicapped by illness, injury or congenital deformity or such disability as may be prescribed'.

This clearly reflects the medical model dominant at the time.

Historically as reflects the terms used, children with disabilities were seen to a degree with prejudice and unacceptability and as a source of amusement (Warner 2006). Quality of life and future potential of child or young person with a disability were not seen in a positive light. Society in the main chose to use institutionalised care as a means of managing what was often seen as a problem to society, the same could be said historically of individuals with mental health issues.

The history of this field is explored in some depth by Atkinson *et al.* (1997) who present both the picture of institutionalised care and examples of individuals living in community settings although in the minority. Children were frequently removed from their families at birth often on the advice of health or social care professionals on the presumption that families would not be able to manage their child's care. Warner (2006) writes of the notion of 'personal tragedy' on the birth of such a child, which sadly still abounds today. The separation of children from their families to institutions where their families were not able to visit or had limited visiting opportunities (Atkinson *et al.* 1997) resulted in children being brought up in an impersonal manner by their custodians, lacking the care and love that a family might offer. Although there are some environments and communities where children with learning disabilities were an integral part of the community, Atkinson *et al.* (1997) gives some examples of this, and in particular some more rural communities have in general had a more inclusive approach than has been observed in other areas at the same time.

The impetus for change from a place where large residential institutions were the norm came from social scientists in the 1950s in favour of smaller more community-based homes where social intellectual and emotional benefits were demonstrated. There were also moves to residential schools or even special communities for individuals with specific learning needs or physical disabilities where normality within a secure environment is promoted.

Over the past 20 years, further changes supported by the Children's Act (1989) and the Welfare of Children in Hospital (DH 1991) in recognition that children are best cared for at home. The central aim of the Community Care Act (1990) was to provide the necessary support structures to enable people to live in their own homes. The 10,989 white paper caring for people confirmed the government to move to centralise services for local health and social care provision and a reduction in isolated institutionalised care to a position where children with disabilities are supported to live with their families. Recent figures suggest that 90% of children with disabilities now live with their families (CAF 2007). Such changes have thus necessitated changes in the way services have been organised; the need for residential institutions and traditional 'Children's Homes' has reduced in favour of respite services (short breaks) away from home and support packages for families to continue to care for their child at home.

With regard to education there, children with disabilities are often educated in schools with specially trained staff and facilities which are suited to children with significant disabilities. Recently, policy focusing on inclusion (Gibson and McGahren 2001) has made increased efforts made for children disabilities to attend main stream schools with support rather than be excluded (Moving to Mainstream 1998). Examples of children with Down's syndrome or children with disabilities such as attention deficit hyperactivity disorder (ADHD) and autism can be accommodated within some main stream schools. However, there continues to be some debate around such issues, particularly in relation to the provision of adequate resources and preparation of main stream schools to support children and young people with disabilities (David *et al.* 1997) in mainstream education.

Changes in the attitudes of society have probably also affected the way in which children and young people with learning difficulties are viewed and treated to a 'more enlightened approach' (Warner 2006). Although families still experience considerable difficulties in the support available from the community and statutory services, *Valuing People* (DH 2005) highlights current difficulties in providing resources and services. A number of organisations provide support for families with disabilities both physically and promoting the cause of such families; these include Contact a Family, Leonard Cheshire, Council for Disabled Children, The Disabled living Foundation and many other specific disability groups.

The current sphere of disability nursing

Current policy in particular the National Service Framework (NSF) for children (DFES 2004a), *Every Child Matters* (DFES 2003a) and Disability Partnership have all argued for a more co-ordinated approach for families with children who have disabilities and complex needs. They require that commissioning bodies change the way that children's services are organised and similarly provide for easier access for families to access a range of services, thus many UK wide project groups who are working towards children's trusts. There is also a need for more joined up working between health, social care and education to reflect both the needs of families and the principles underlying *Every Child Matters* (DFES 2003a) relating to shared information and safeguarding children who, many of whom, are known to be in need (Crosse 1992).

Policy influences

National Service framework for Children, Young People and Maternity Services (2004a) – Standard 8
National Service Framework for Mental Health (1999)
Youth Matters (2005)
Every Child Matters (2003a)
CAMHS Grant (2003–2004)
Valuing People (DH 2001)
The Children Act 2004
Special Educational Needs and Disability Act 2001
Disability Discrimination Act 2005

The focus of many of the aforementioned policies indicate that there needs to be a change in essence from services that traditionally have not worked so closely together and a change in emphasis towards partnership and valuing the individual child and their family unit. However, achieving such changes could be seem to be problematic for some services. The management and provision of disability services across the country varies greatly (Audit Commission 2003).

And there continues to be some debate around where services should be located as far as commissioning and management and location, although as discussed earlier, UK-wide partnership projects have paved the way in many ways to more co-ordinated working. Traditionally, services for children and young people with disabilities have been situated in social care settings, and it is unusual to have such services located or offered specifically in health care settings. Nationally, children's disability services have often been managed as part of an adult learning disability team and not necessarily integrated with other children's health services. Although children's services within social and health care are often separated, there is much joint working between paediatric community nurses and children's learning disability (LD) community nurses. Working closely with education is also very important as education is the work of children, and they spend a great deal of their day at school.

There is much overlap in what support children and young people and their families require as few children have a single defined disability, many children have some physical disability, some have complex needs and some do not have a clearly diagnosed syndrome or medical condition. Consequently, it is often difficult to and not appropriate to separate the care that such children needs different services and to different practitioners. Watson *et al.* (2002) supports this notion that children with complex needs have the same range of needs as other disabled children in addition to technical and medical support. One model of care is not sufficient; children require a person-centred holistic approach to care.

As discussed earlier, efforts should be made to co-ordinate services, so that as far as possible they reduce the stress and difficulties of families with different professionals. There have been examples of families having to seek information and support from a number of different services, including those that support the child's health care needs, social services and education needs. This can result in families attending appointments on several different dates' in different locations, with no clear co-ordination. As Watson *et al.* (2002) describes, it is not always clear whose role is to provide support for families, in particular those with complex needs; this can result in the onus on the family to liaise between upwards of six services. Professionals working with the child and family may include:

- Children's disability nurse and community workers.
- Social worker.
- Therapists such as physiotherapist, occupational therapists, speech and language.
- Special educational need co-ordinator and teachers.

For some children and families who require funded packages of care, there should be some negotiation as to the sources of funding depending on a particular child's needs and also how that package is delivered. These packages often evolve over time as the child's needs change; thus, care co-ordination is an important factor in supporting such families (Sloper 1999).

Specific services for individuals with disabilities particularly learning disabilities are often not necessarily orientated within children's services, and this can make the co-ordination of care packages difficult. Greco and Sloper (2004) discuss the importance of the key worker scheme in co-coordinating care for the child with disabilities and their family. A specific aspect of the role of the practitioner is to liaise with other services that the child or young person comes into contact with and that may be the acute hospital setting when a child becomes unwell, with other therapists, with schools, families and other carers. There may be similar issues where a young person is to make the transition to adult disability services where liaison is needed to ensure that the transition to the adult service usually located in social care is smooth.

Currently, services reflect the need for community-based support for many families, although there is still a need for respite care (short breaks) for children and young people. It is also an issue that a notable proportion of children with some disabilities are 'looked after' in some form, in foster care, residential school or in the private sector. For some children with severe disabilities or challenging learning, their families are unable or find it very difficult to manage their child at home in the long term; consequently, some or all of their care is provided away from home.

It is also the case that children with disabilities who have complex physical needs as Watson *et al.* (2002) explores require services where their carers can receive the support that they need in an appropriate environment which is often at home, although the provision of such a service is not without its problems. Consequently, it is not possible to assume that all children and young people can be supported entirely with community-based resources. Provision for acutely ill children, families who cannot care for their child at home and for children and families who need to spend some time apart needs to be provided. Hence, the need for a diverse range of services and roles to support children and young people with disabilities and examples of services across the country are easily accessed through an Internet search of 'Children and Disabilities'.

Case study: Children's disability service Stockport

One such service based in Stockport in the North West is physically and strategically located within children's services located in an acute health care setting and managed within the local children's partnership. The service is co-ordinated from the base within the children's centre from where child and adolescent mental health service, community nursing, acute in-patient services and therapy services are also offered.

The children's disability service is co-ordinated by a clinical nurse specialist and offers a community-based service, short breaks, palliative care and a child development unit. It also offers care co-ordination and supports the delivery of packages of care for children with complex needs.

It has advantages in its hospital location in having access to key medical consultants and acute services. Although its location can mean that children with a disability are seen in a medical environment, some children find the 'hospital environment' and 'uniforms' worn by some professionals frightening. Social care workers and adult learning disability service and other partnerships are located elsewhere.

Case studies from individuals working within some of these services are given as an illustration.

Skills for supporting children and their families with disabilities

Children's nurses have not traditionally followed a career pathway into the field of children with disabilities; however, this does not mean that children's nurses are restricted from working in those settings. There is a diverse range of roles that are developing in areas where children with disabilities and complex needs are cared for (see also Learning Disability Networks 2007) such that they are open to a range of practitioners with backgrounds in nursing, public health, education and social care backgrounds. This is also reflected in the current pre-registration Learning Disability Nursing courses that are expanding to incorporate a social work qualification, reflecting the need for a joined up approach to individuals with learning.

The growing diversity in Learning Disability Nursing and the new broader definition of children with disabilities has demonstrated a need for equally diverse skills that will be explored later, particularly as the philosophy towards family-orientated care predominates, as Warner (2006) describes 'building relationships' with families is a vital part of the role. Key skills for professionals working with children as outlined in the earlier chapters as indicated by the Nursing and Midwifery Council (NMC), and the common skills of the Department of Education and Skills (DFES) indicate that those trained in children's nursing together with other professionals would be required to demonstrate a level of competency in these as a base line to other key skill sets.

Attending to the basic physical needs of children and young people with a learning disability is a key aspect of working with children with disabilities, and as children with complex needs are supported more in the community, there has been a greater emphasis for the nursing staff to demonstrate competence in more technological skills such as respiratory support, airway support such as tracheostomy and feeding through nasogastric or gastrostomy, and commonly, this is combined with both the need to offer support and to some degree educate families in these skills once seen as within the nursing domain.

Skills in promoting appropriate social behaviour and dealing with challenging behaviour are essential to the role of professionals working with children with disabilities. Bernal (2006) notes that a significant proportion of children may exhibit difficult or challenging behaviour for many reasons. Professionals working in the field need to develop skills in both understanding these types of behaviour and responding to it. Nurses or other professionals may lie in setting up and supporting behavioural programmes for families, desensitisation programmes or running courses for parents with children with behavioural issues such as Webster Stratton. The role could also be to support other health professionals in acute settings in managing difficult behaviour or supporting children and young people in their homes.

Supporting communication skills for children and families is paramount. Warner (2006) describes how the practitioner can support language development where possible but in particular assisting children and their families in communicating together using other methods where a child does not have fluent language or speech. Total communication is an approach to communication that makes use of a number of modes of communication such as signed or auditory, written and visual. What you use will be dependant on the needs and abilities of the child (Meyer and Lowerbrau 1990). Total communication is about communicating in any way you can. It is not just about talking, but it is about signing, pointing to pictures, symbols, photographs or objects. It is also about using gesture or body movement.

These can include helping children, families and those working with them in using communication aids both low tech such as pointer boards, signing and tactile systems or high tech such as computers and voice readers. Clearly, the support of speech and language therapists is also important in this aspect.

Supporting families whose children have physical and behavioural or developmental needs is again a crucial aspect of disability nursing, and consequently, the ability to support families emotionally is a significant skill required of those working in this field. In particular, the partnership aspects are outlined by Smith *et al.* (2002) and Hutchfield (1999). Well-developed listening skills are an important part of the relationship building that has been mentioned earlier.

Co-ordination of services and support packages of care needed for children and young people with disabilities is a complex skill and involves liaising with acute care settings, working with a team providing services for a child from short breaks to complex packages of care provided in the community. This can also involve acting as a key worker or lead professional for a child or young person and reviewing progress with a team of other professionals although as Greco and Sloper (2004) indicate provision of such schemes is variable across the country as is the degree of multi-agency involvement in overseeing services.

Multidisciplinary working is also important in managing the transition to adult services as Thulgate (2006) describes. Education, career, health, independence, family and living and resources are all important components to consider in the overall plan, and this approach is also reflected in the children's NSF (DFES 2004a). Liaison between other professionals in schools is important to support a child's education and provide consistency in the behavioural and social skill development.

There is also a need to work with therapists to support ongoing work and contribute to overall assessments of children with other therapists and professionals.

Educational aspects of the role are a growing area, and often, there is a need to provide services that can advise parents on problems such as supporting healthy eating and managing obesity, sleep programmes, social skills and issues around expressing sexuality. This aspect of the role may require the practitioner to take further training to support their knowledge in a particular area. There appears to be a growing awareness that in order for children and young people to learn to function independently in society, issues around sexuality and sexual health need to be addressed, and families are also recognising this need.

Play development work is another part of enabling children and young people to fulfil their potential. Warner describes how play can enhance children's development in many areas such as physical, cognitive, social and emotional aspects. It is also important to recognise the importance of play as the normal part of the social life of a child or young person with or without a disability. It can also support peer and family attachment and relationships.

Training

Health professionals from nursing backgrounds who work with children with disabilities do not necessarily follow generic learning disability training or necessarily all have similar backgrounds.

A review of staff working with children with a range of physical, learning and developmental disabilities would reveal that a number of staff are trained in Learning Disability Nursing and a proportion with a learning disability and social work qualification at diploma or degree level. Others may have qualifications in children's nursing, school nursing or health visiting. Previously, nursing staff may have held a RGN or RNMH mental handicap qualification.

Provision of post qualification courses varies greatly but may be tailored to suit the specific area that the practitioner is working in, such as community, palliative care or short breaks/respite, public health, complex needs – children's nursing. Although partly because of the diversity of the field, there are often difficulties in accessing appropriate courses because of the lack of provision or not being considered appropriate for disability nurses. Examples or post qualification courses accessed by practitioners in the field include courses related to:

- Mental health issues.
- Dealing with challenging behaviour/behavioural management.
- MA or PG certification in profound learning disability.
- Community specialist practitioner.
- Children with high dependency needs.
- Family planning.
- Play development.
- Parenting – Webster Stratton.
- Continence.

Examples from practitioners working with children and families with disabilities

The child development team

The role of the practitioner working in this area would usually include children who are in the younger age range and would need some very different skills. In some services, the assessment and support of young children with developmental needs is located within a health visiting or another service not necessarily linked to a children's disability services. Similarly, the role of the nurse or practitioner working in a child development team may be from a health visiting, school nurse or children's nursing background. In a service based in Stockport, the senior practitioner who co-ordinates the service has a background in children's nursing but has also worked as a community children's nurse and a school nurse in a special school before taking on this role.

Working in this area requires the practitioner to provide early support for families whose child has a diagnosis of a condition requiring long-term support to assist the child reach his potential. Children may reach an early diagnosis in the case of Down's syndrome or similar congenital conditions, whereas others may be diagnosed following assessment over time, as in the cases of autism or cerebral palsy. Although there are also groups of children who present with a global developmental delay which following assessment and screening do not have a specific diagnosis condition but nevertheless require support and information in the long term.

Skills in communication with families are imperative not only in both listening and helping in the assessment process but also in giving of information, which can often be difficult time for families. Boster and Warner (2006) stress the importance of delivering the diagnosis, the manner that it is given and information required by families. During the past 10 years, the importance on giving the diagnosis in an appropriate manner has been recognised, and there is clear guidance available (RCN 1999, DH 2003, www.rightfromthestart.org) for best practice, and practitioners are required to be competent 'sharing the news' alongside medical professionals who often make the final diagnosis.

The practitioner as part of the assessment process should have a good knowledge of normal child development and factors that may influence this. The service in Stockport usually conducts an assessment session following referral to the service. This session allows all members of the Multidisciplinary team (MDT) an opportunity to make their assessment, who then meet to combine their assessments before a feedback meeting within 3–5 weeks where findings are explained to the family. In the case of autism, a diagnosis can usually be given on the same morning, the earliest age that autism can be diagnosed is ~2.5 years. The senior practitioner would also chair key meetings where new cases are accepted and recent cases are reviewed. The child development unit offers with regular therapy sessions and group sessions for particular groups of families and play sessions, and the practitioner has a key role in organising and facilitating such sessions.

A key element to the role of the practitioner working in the child development service is co-ordination and liaison with the multidisciplinary team, who usually includes lead paediatricians, educational psychologists, occupational therapists, physiotherapists, speech and language therapists and nursery nurses. Such services often include close links with portage services and care co-ordination where key workers are organised to support specific families. Senior practitioners would also act as a key worker to a number of families.

Secondary care

Acute liaison

Children with disabilities frequently require admission to acute children's services due to physical or social reasons, and there are very few specially designed units in the country that can specifically cater for children and their families who have complex physical needs who have disabilities. A four-bedded unit in Manchester located within an acute National Health Service (NHS) trust opened 25 years ago offers this type of support and can also offer respite for children with very complex needs. Where such a service is not available, there is often a need for support and advice for nursing and medical staff in acute areas in caring for children with disabilities.

Often, the dependency of children with complex needs means that they cannot be adequately supported in an acute children's ward without the presence of their family or main carer.

The nature of support may be related to technical clinical skills relating to tracheostomy care and managing feeding. These may also relate to more complex issues such as managing complex seizures, moving and positioning a child with complex needs. Nursing staff may also need advice in how to communicate with the non-verbal child and especially in the recognition of pain and responsiveness.

Support offered in these situations may be offered by way of the children's disability team or a nurse specialist in a specific area. Children with disabilities who have complex needs may also have specific needs which may draw on the skills of a play therapist and other staff experienced in supporting developmental and educational stimulation.

Community work: case study

Children's community learning disability nurse

My interest in working with people led me towards a psychology degree on leaving Sixth Form College. I studied in London and on graduating began working as an occupational therapy assistant. This gave me firsthand experience of working in a large organisation and built on my previous experience working on summer play schemes for young adults with a learning disability.

Occupational therapy work provided an excellent opportunity to develop relationship building skills because of the close client contact it involved. After 18 months, I felt it was time to move away from London and began to work as a senior support worker in a home treatment service. This involved working with people with severe and enduring mental health difficulties. I worked alongside qualified nurses in a challenging community setting. The variety of the work and the varied demands on my time meant that no 2 days were the same. Assisting individuals and families through difficult times proved highly rewarding and laid the foundations for my desire to gain qualified status.

I joined the joint programme at Manchester and Salford University where I was trained in social work and learning disability nursing. This intensive and thought-provoking course provided placements as well as theoretical challenges.

I have been employed for the past 5 years as a children's community learning disability nurse within a small team of community nurses and support workers. My role is extremely varied, and each day will bring different demands and experiences.

Children on my caseload will have moderate to severe learning disabilities; I work with the child themselves and the family/carers dependent on individual need. A predominant part of my role is to provide emotional support to families during times of crisis or general difficulty; I regularly liaise and refer to multi-agency services such as social care, sibling support and welfare benefits.

The team provides behaviour management advice to encourage positive patterns of behaviour within the home environment; this involves regular liaison with the child's education setting to ensure consistency of care. We support families to identify triggers to specific behaviours, set realistic behavioural goals and to find specific motivational rewards for the child. Families are supported either on a 1:1 basis or through a positive parenting group which I co-facilitate with my colleagues.

We offer a 'Social Skills Group' to young people aged 12–16 years. The course content will vary dependent on individual need but concentrates on reducing vulnerability, that is encourages stranger danger, personal hygiene, and body awareness. Each course promotes social development and friendships through group games and activities. I will often offer individual follow-up sessions. When young people require additional input, this may include self-esteem building, anger management and keeping safe.

I am regularly involved in Play Development Groups that encourage social interaction skills for children under the age of 6 years. Each group is structured and follows a visual timetable. My role is to encourage play skills such as turn taking, sharing and waiting through the medium of play.

All individual work with children/young adults will very often require specific visual systems to support individual learning styles. My role therefore is to devise appropriate materials to enable individuals to engage in activities where possible. Interventions need to be adapted, so that children can be included where possible.

Much of my assessment work involves observations of children in differing environmental settings as well as close liaison with significant others. This helps to build a wider picture of the child's development.

Owing to my varied role, it is important that I identify training needs for myself and have access to regular supervision. I supervise support staff and help to manage the team through rota systems.

The role is challenging yet rewarding and provides a balance of experiences between family work, direct work with children and liaison with professionals from multi-agency teams.

Susie Tinsley

Respite/short breaks services

The current philosophy with regard to respite care or often known as short breaks is not just to 'give parents a break'; it may also give parents time to spend with other siblings, who are often seen as being disadvantaged. Respite can promote independence for the child or young person with specific learning disabilities. As a child develops, they would normally start to spend periods of time away from home, and one of the aims of the service is to offer such children with learning disabilities the opportunity to gain independence and spend time with other children, developing communication skills and social skills through play and other activities. The opportunity allows some integration and the ability to develop social skills away from home. Thulgate *et al.* (2006) explores the benefits and organisation of respite services in more detail, although as McConkey and Adams (2000) and Treneman *et al.* (1997) indicate that demand for such services is high and provision is not sufficient for many families.

Case study

Short breaks service: staff nurse

Before undertaking my training between the ages of 16 and 18, I worked with children with learning disabilities on holiday play schemes where I became interested in learning disability nursing. I then took a year out after A level then commenced the diploma in learning disability nursing at Sheffield. I then worked for a year with adults with learning disabilities, gaining valuable experience and confidence. I moved to Stockport in 1996 to work in a unit for children with learning disabilities. I also worked with children and their families in a community setting. I am currently working in a purpose built unit for children with learning disability receiving respite care.

A typical day – or not

Each day is not typical as it involves different approaches to working in the day time, evenings, weekends or school holidays.

In general, key aspects of the role include caring for the children and ensuring that they are safe and secure and meeting their basic needs. Play is a particularly important aspect of the work, as children need 'normal' stimulation when in the unit, such as physical play 'rough and tumble' watching TV, games, art activities and utilising the sensory room and promoting relaxation.

I also ensure that prescribed medication is administered.

During a school day, after the early morning rush to get all the children up and ready for school, once the children have been collected, there are other important aspects to the role.

This can range from staff/student supervision, staff meetings, rota planning, home visits to meet new children and existing families.

Other work includes updating care plans, visiting children in schools to get an insight into behaviours at school and liaising with the multidisciplinary team.

General house upkeep also needs to be done such as ordering meals and equipment and ensuring cleaning and tidying takes place.

The majority of children have a diagnosis of autism spectrum disorder (ASD) with associated severe learning disabilities and challenging behaviour. These children require more structure although this is not a school environment, and the unit aims to be a home from home; thus, it is more relaxed. We aim to offer choice and promote independence. Other children have severe physical disabilities and require feeding (orally or through gastrostomy and Nasogastric tube).

All activities and care need risk assessing for moving and handling.

We work closely with parents to continue caring for their child was they would be cared for at home. We write up their care plans with the parents in order for consistency of care from home to the unit. Within each profile is a comprehensive risk assessment.

All meals are provided by the unit unless they are on strict diets; then parents send in their food. Food is all child friendly and prepared by the staff which promotes choice rather than just providing hospital food.

Packages are put together from health, but if there are additional needs (require more support), then assessments are carried out by social services and ourselves for funding to be made available for one to one support.

James Collier

Support for children with life-limiting conditions

A number of children's disability teams or community children's teams are now offering specific services for children with life-limiting and life-threatening conditions. As mentioned previously, there are increasing efforts to enable families to care for their child at home, and this may be in actual physical support of nurses or carers in the home. Such services also work with various agencies to assist the family and provide information and advice to the family and other workers. Emotional support for the family including the siblings is also offered together with specific support following the loss of a child.

Many of these services are new and reflecting hospice services. They may not be fully funded by the statutory agencies or they may be funded by interim projects or charities such as the Lottery Fund or the new opportunities fund.

Nurses working in this field may also come from a range of backgrounds including children's nursing, palliative care hospice care and cancer nursing backgrounds.

Senior roles

The nurse working in a senior position with teams caring for children with disabilities may have a background in adult disability nursing, children's disability, community nursing or public health. This background may relate to the particular service offered or the interest of the individual.

Key aspects of the role currently reflect the need to promote the strategic direction of services fitting with health and social care economy and, additionally, helping to further the development of the children's agenda (see NSF) and supporting the business plan for the children and young people's partnership.

Service evaluation is increasing in importance especially in reflecting the changing needs of its users. It is important that someone is responsible for the delivery of social care packages at a senior level form the service.

As in other senior positions, the manager is responsible for ensuring that teams have adequate staff to maintain the service either responding to short-term staffing issues or in recruiting and forming business plans for the teams and ensuring quality and performance reviews integral to the above.

Financial management of local budget would also be integral to the role. Other aspects of the role may include introducing the common assessment framework and working on project groups' transition groups.

The future

The future of the field of children's disability nursing seems to be that disability will be seen as a broader field of care and that learning disability, sensory disability, complex needs, behavioural problems and children with life-limited illnesses will not be seen in separate services and specialities. There are currently strategic moves toward more joined up working, seeing learning, social and sensory disability and the affect on the family unit and maximising the potential for individual children with disabilities. The work towards achieving children and young people trusts should continue following some of the earlier partnership projects between health, social care and education.

The introduction of core skills (DFES 2007) will be continue to be reflected in teams working with children and young people with disability together with the common assessment framework.

Following the area of transition to adult services has also begun to be more significant issue, and this type of work is still evolving.

References

Atkinson D, Jackson M. and Walmsley J (1997). *Forgotten Lives – Exploring the History of Learning Disability*. Plymouth: British Institute of Learning Disabilities.

Audit Commission (2003). *Services for Disabled Children – A Review of Services for Disabled Children and Their Families*. Audit Commission, London.

Bernal C (2006). Challenging the 'tragedy', Chapter 3 in Warner H (2006). *Meeting the Needs of Children with Disabilities, Families and Professionals Facing the Challenge Together*. London: Routledge.

Boster K and Warner H (2006). Getting it right – the initial diagnosis, Chapter 5 in Warner H (2006). *Meeting the Needs of Children with Disabilities, Families and professionals Facing the Challenge Together*. London: Routledge.

Committee of the Central Health Services Council (1959). *The Welfare of Children in Hospital (Platt Report)*. London: HMSO.

Contact a Family (CAF) (2007). Contact a family factsheet: About families with disabilities. www.cafamily.org.uk/students (accessed 14 June 2007).

Crosse S, Kaye E and Ratnofsky A (1992). *A Report on the Maltreatment of Children with Disabilities – National Center on Child Abuse and Neglect Administration on Children*. US Department of Health and Human Services, Washington DC.

David T, Moir J and Herbert E (1997). Curriculum issues in early childhood: Implications for families. In: Carpenter B (ed.), *Families in Context*. London: David Fulton.

Department of Education and Skills (DFES) (2003a). *Every Child Matters*. Nottingham: DFES.

Department of Education and Skills (DFES) (2004a). *Disabled Children and Young People and Those with Complex Health Needs – The National Service Framework for Children, Young People and Maternity Services – Standard 8*. Department of Health, London.

Department of Education and Skills (DFES) (2004b). *Core Standards – National Service Framework for Children, Young People and Maternity Services*. Department of Health, London.

Department of Education and Skills (DFES) (2007). www.dfes.gov.uk/commoncore (accessed July 2007).

Department of Health (DH) (1989). *The Children's Act. An Introductory Guide for the NHS*. London: HMSO.

Department of Health (DH) (1991). *Welfare of Children in Hospital*. London: Her Majesty's Stationery Office.

Department of Health (DH) (1998). *Moving to Mainstream: The Report of a National Inspection of Services for Adults with Learning Disabilities*. London: HMSO.

Department of Health (DH) (1999). *National Service Framework for Mental Health: Modern Standards and Service Models*. London: DH.

Department of Health (DH) (2001). *Valuing People – A New Strategy for Learning Disability for the 21st Century*. DH, Washington DC.

Department of Health (DH), Scope (2003). *Right from the Start Template: Good practice in sharing the News, DH: Scope in partnership with the Right from the Start Working Group.* www.rightfromthestart.org.

Department of Health (DH) (2005). *The Government's Annual Report on Learning Disability 2005*. Norwich, HMSO.

Gibson C and McGahren Y (2001). *When Your Child has Special Needs: A Guide for Parents Who Care for a Child with a Disability, Special Needs or Rare Disorder*. London: Contact a Family.

Greco V and Sloper P (2004). Care co-ordination and key worker schemes for disabled children: Results of a UK-wide survey. *Child: Care, Health and Development*, 30, 13–20.

HMSO (2005). *Youth Matters*. Norwich: HMSO.

Hutchfield K (1999). Family centred care: A concept analysis. *Journal of Advanced Nursing*, 29(5), 1178–1187.

Learning Disability Networks (2007). www.learningdisabilites.org.uk (accessed April 2007).

Meyer P and Lowenbraun S (1990) Total communication use among elementary teachers of hearing-impaired children. *American Annals of the Deaf*, 135, 257–263.

McConkey R and Adams L (2000). Matching short break services for children with learning disabilities to family needs and preferences. *Child: Care, Health and Development*, 25(5), 429–444.

National Health Service and Community Care Act (1990). Crown Copyright 1990.

Northfield (2003). *What is learning disability* on NHS National Electronic Library for Health (NeLH). http://libraries.nelh.uklearningdisabilities/viewResource.asp?uri=http//libraries,nelh.nhs.uk/common/resources/?id=31736.

Royal College of Nursing (RCN) (1999) *Supporting Families when They are Told of Their Child's Health Disorder or Disability*. London: RCN.

Sloper (1999). Models of service support for patients of disabled children. What do we know? What do we need to know? *Child Health Care and Development*, 24(2), 85–99.

Smith L, Coleman V and Bradshaw M (2002). *Family-Centred Care: Concept, Theory and Practice*. London: Palgrave.

Thompson (2003). *Promoting Equality: Challenging Discrimination and Oppression*, 2nd edn. Basingstoke: Macmillan.

Thulgate C (2006). The importance of appropriate respite care, Chapter 12 in Warner H (2006). *Meeting the Needs of Children with Disabilities, Families and Professionals Facing the Challenge Together*. London: Routledge.

Treneman M, Corkery A, Dowdney L and Hammond J (1997). Respite-care needs – met and unmet: Assessment of needs for children with disability. *Developments in Medical Neurology*, 39(8), 548–553.

Warner H (2006). *Meeting the Needs of Children with Disabilities, Families and Professionals Facing the Challenge Together*. London: Routledge.

Watson D, Townsley R and Abbott D (2002). Exploring multi-agency working in services to disabled children with complex healthcare needs and their families. *Journal of Clinical Nursing*, 11, 367–375.

Chapter 9
Safeguarding and Supporting Children and Young People and Their Families

Hazel Chamberlain

A shared responsibility and the need for effective working between agencies and professionals that have different roles and expertise are required if children are to be protected from harm and their welfare promoted.

(Department of Education and Skills 2006b, p. 10)

This chapter explores the role of nursing in safeguarding children and young people, their working with other agencies such as education, social work and police and the policy that has influenced those practices.

The concept of childhood and the rights of children within the British society has received increased recognition from health and welfare services during the past 50 years. The need to demonstrate, by those professional groups, that the philosophy of care for children and families incorporates a recognition of those rights, and furthermore underpins their practice with children and young people, has served to bring about a concept of family-centred care throughout that period.

Child rearing practices have changed too. What was once considered to be acceptable means of controlling or disciplining of children by adults, who were responsible for their care, has been questioned. This has resulted in the lowering of thresholds of the definition of what constitutes child abuse within the society (DH 1995; Parton *et al.* 1997) and has lead to legislation of ensuring that the rights of children and young people are reflected by all members of that society in the UK. In the updated Children Act 2004, the five outcomes – right to be healthy, to stay safe, to make a positive contribution, to receive education and to achieve economic well-being as an adult – have been incorporated, with those agencies that provide services to children and young people being held to account and deliver appropriate services to enable children and young people to achieve. These outcomes apply for services offered to all children regardless of the cultural or economic background of their family.

The abuse of children is no new phenomenon. Within the UK, the Liverpool Society for the Prevention of Child Cruelty (NSPCC 2004) was established as an organisation in 1884, being developed to meet the needs of children who were living in poverty and neglect. This is now known as the charity NSPCC. There are also examples from literature throughout time that reflect the perceptions of acceptable parenting practices at that time (De Mause 1974). In the latter part of the 20th century, the study of Caffey (1946) identified unexplained fractures in children at post-mortem examination, and the subsequent publication by Kempe *et al.* (1962) 'The Battered Baby Syndrome' demonstrated that some children were being killed or severely injured by their parents. These publications influenced practitioners such as paediatricians and social workers to follow a medical model of child abuse with the emphasis on the presence of physical injury to the child being a prerequisite to demonstrate that the child was suffering harm. In the mid-1970s in the UK, after the public inquiry into the death of Maria Colwell (1974), a framework was developed, which essentially encouraged practitioners, working in child care, to assess the context in which children lived by identifying risk factors that could subject them to harm within that family setting.

During the 1990s, the shift from child abuse as a medical model to that of it being a 'socially constructive phenomenon' (Gibbons *et al.* 1995b) was developing with recognition that health, education and social needs of children and young people were more intertwined and that it was the context in which the child lived that needed to be assessed. In the UK, this lead to government policies based on the principle that early intervention with families prevented the risk of child abuse (DH 1998). A multi-agency assessment tool, the purpose of which was to aid the assessment of families, to create a common ground between professionals from different agencies, who were involved in the assessment process and to reduce conflict, was developed. The tool was also aimed at reducing multiple assessments of families with the objective of reducing the number of times the families were asked by the multi-agency team to provide information (DH 2000a).

Subsequent reports such as the Bristol Royal Infirmary (Department of Health 2001), the Joint Inspectors Report (DFES 2002) and the Inquiry into the death of Victoria Climbié (Laming 2003) influenced the development of guidance programmes such as the Every Child Matters (DFES 2004) and the National Service Framework for Children, Young people and Maternity Services (DFES 2004). These ensured that safeguarding of children's welfare was considered especially by public sector organisations that were responsible for delivery of services to all children and families. The subsequent updated Children Act 2004 further incorporated safeguarding of children and young people by changing the principles identified within stated documents into a recognised legislative framework for practice of health and welfare professionals.

Since 1995, Department of Health guidance (DH 1995, 1999, DFES 2006b) stated the need for each health organisation, including hospitals, to identify a lead nurse and/or a midwife and a lead doctor to ensure that health employees of each organisation were able to access advice when dealing with a child or young person who may have suffered child abuse. The lead professionals were also charged with ensuring that those employees had access to training to inform their practice. They were also responsible to Local Authority Area Child Protection Committees to undertake serious case reviews under Chapter 8 of the government guidance (DH 1995, 1999, DFES 2006b).

In community health care settings, these roles appeared to be well defined, with health visiting seen as the key health group delivering child protection services. This was comparative to acute trusts where the lead nurse role was often taken as 'add on' for senior nurses, often nurse managers of children's units, to undertake. Although this situation in some acute hospital settings persists, there is an increasing drive to develop the role of the safeguarding children's nurse by employing full-time nurses within acute health organisations.

Senior nurses for child protection in community and those in acute trusts clearly supported the belief that child abuse was most commonly initially identified by a family's health visitor, who delivered a universal health service to all children and families, coupled with the view point that very few children suffering or at risk of suffering from child abuse ever visited hospitals.

The role of the safeguarding children's nurse requires a sufficient seniority to provide strategic overview for each trust on the service provision necessary to ensure that children and young people's needs are met and comply with the current government guidance. Until the early 2000s, the role of the safeguarding children's nurse, in both hospital and community health care settings, was very much focused on the needs of children and young people who were likely or who had actually suffered child abuse.

Since the Victoria Climbié Inquiry (2003), the need for acute health trusts to develop more robust structures to address child protection and safeguarding of children and young people within their organisations has identified that the abuse of some children and young people has been identified at hospital visits, commonly when the child presents with other health issues (see Case Scenario 1).

Case Scenario 1

Kyle is 3 weeks old. He attends the Accident and Emergency Department with symptoms of bronchiolitis. When a chest X-ray is performed, fractures to three ribs are found. Referral was made to social services and police on advice from the safeguarding children's nurse, and further information was sought from other professionals such as health visitor so that practitioners had more information with respect to the context in which Kyle and his family lived.

Furthermore, the perception of health staff as to what constitutes an abusive act or is recognised as a risk to the child's welfare has widened. The needs of children with disability, chronic or complex health needs has been considered under the auspice of the safeguarding agenda (Kennedy and Wonnacott 2005). The effectiveness of nurses in safeguarding of children and young people is dependent on robust assessment of children, including assessment of the effects of ill health on the family unit and the ability of the family to cope.

In some acute hospital trusts children and young people may not have discrete health service provision and may receive health care within a clinical setting designed to meet the health needs of adults, but are treated (this includes young people of 16–18 years receiving health services), the safeguarding nurse ensures that health staff, whose main focus of care is to adult patients, receive training in safeguarding of children and young people. Health practitioners are asked to particularly question parenting capacity of adult patients, who present to health disciplines with key risk factors for families such as domestic violence, drug and alcohol use and mental health issues. Section 10 of the Children Act 2004 places an onus on health trusts to ensure that effective reporting of concerns about a child's welfare is made by practitioners caring for adult patients.

Competencies to demonstrate the ability of all health trusts, including ambulance trusts, to safeguard children and young people are inspected by the Health Care Commission, and the health trusts receive rating on the organisation's compliance with those competencies (Standards for Better Health 2005).

Multi-agency working, conflict and partnership with families

The first public enquiry in the UK into the death of a child from physical abuse (Ministry of Health 1945, see Home Office 1945), and numerous subsequent inquiries, have identified that one of the biggest risk factors for the failure to protect vulnerable children and young people, by agencies, has been the seeming inability to work together. This has ultimately contributed to negative outcomes of intervention for children and families (Hallett and Birchall 1995, Reder *et al.* 1998). A number of factors that compromise effective working together have been identified. These include the inability of individual agencies to understand the role of others, power struggles between agencies and the differences in perceptions of risk by individual workers carrying out the assessment of risk to children and families. Laming (2003) points out the amount of time the health staff spent making assessments of what is needed to be done to safeguard a child, but then those identified tasks were not completed as there was no clear delegation. There was no system in place which reviewed that planned action for safeguarding children and young people had been carried out. This ultimately results in no action for families.

A key factor resulting in effective outcomes for children and families is effective assessment and case planning. Both local and national reviews of cases in the 1980s and 1990s in the UK identified the need for multi-agency assessment of an individual family's needs to be made rather than that based on the assessment of one agency i.e. social services with the result that there would be shared assessment and shared accountability of decisions made (Bridge Childcare Consultancy 1995, Laming 2003).

In 2000, the DH in UK published guidance for all health and welfare professionals in the Framework for Assessment of Children and Families. Its intent was that this framework would be used by all agencies that carried out assessments of any child in any situation. It placed the child as the focus for assessment and encouraged the practitioner to consider three factors in the assessment of all children and young people who were accessing services. These were the need to assess the parent's ability to parent a child, assessment of the context in which the child lived and an assessment of the developmental stage of the child.

The aim of the Assessment Framework (Fig. 9.1) was that the initial assessment would be carried out by the practitioner from whichever agency that had initially made contact with the child, and this was then to be built upon by other practitioners either from that same agency or from others. A key objective to the use of the framework was that more effective assessment would be carried out in the initial stages so that fewer families would need to enter into the child protection process (Gibbons *et al.* 1995a). There was a further improved outcome for families who would not need to keep repeating the same information to practitioners from various agencies and that respect between professionals would be fostered in that the assessment of a professional from one organisation would be accepted by another as being accurate and then built upon and thus reducing

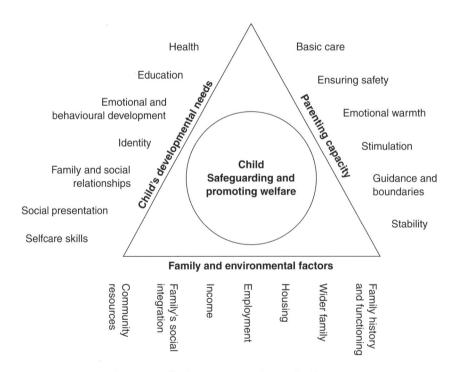

Fig. 9.1   Assessment framework (DH 2000a, p. 89, Appendix A).

conflict. This guidance was to replace the DH's 1988 guidance for assessment, issued only to social service teams with respect to assessment of children and young people.

Since 2000, within health, the framework for assessment of need is used widely for the health assessments of children in the field of health visiting. However, this has not been extended to acute trust nursing assessments of children and young people, which still applies nursing models (Casey 1988, Roper *et al.* 1996) and falls short of considering welfare of children and young people. This has limited the ability of nurses working in acute trusts to recognise and respond to concerns about children and young people's vulnerability.

The lead nurse for safeguarding children will ensure that assessment of the child's social needs is incorporated into assessment of all children in addition to the focus on addressing the physical needs of the child. This has lead to discussion between nursing staff of their failure to document basic information such as what has been discussed with parents, the amount of time that nurses spend speaking with the child or a young person and the need to assess whether a family will be able to cope with the demands placed upon them when a child is diagnosed with ill health or, furthermore, the resources and abilities of the parents and/or child or young person to meet those needs for themselves (Nayda 2004).

Case Scenario 2

A nurse from Accident and Emergency Unit was asked to give evidence in Crown Court with respect to a baby who had suffered sexual abuse. Information in the statement that she presented to the police was not contained in the original documentation made by her on the night which the child was presented. The statement was made 10 days after the child's admission, and the court hearing was 2 years after the event. Her evidence was discredited. It was argued that her documentation at the time of the child's admission did not mirror her police statement. Supervision was sought by the nurse from the child protection team. The nurse spoke to the child protection team of the need to document events outside of the hospital case notes as she was afraid of the risk to her personally from the family and furthermore believed that the information documented by her was inappropriate for submission to hospital case notes.

There is some evidence that when assessment of children and families has been initiated by health professionals, the information shared with other agencies may not be accepted as accurate information resulting in either new assessment being made or the initial assessment being downgraded in importance and the level of risk assessed by the next professional being of lower level. Nayda (2004) states that some nurses may fail to report concerns about the welfare of a child due to their belief that other agencies would not take their concern seriously. Nurses also perceived that an ineffective response from other agencies to the family meant that the nurse's relationship with that family was then damaged. Dale (2004) identified that parents often became aware that there was disagreement between professionals within the multi-agency team, as to the level of risk within their family, and felt that this often had a detrimental effect on the support that they were able to access to meet their family needs. Platt (2006) reviewed 23 case studies of families referred to social services, which bordered on concern to the level of child protection. She then asked social workers, who were involved in the cases, their rationale for the decision making, which subsequently occurred. She concluded that there were five criteria that social workers applied to each case. These were what was the specific harm described for the child, its severity, risk of future harm, parental accountability and whether information was corroborated either by other events or by other professionals. If then there is some breakdown of the way in which information is understood from one professional discipline to another, it is evident that this may ultimately affect the way in which referrals of families into the system is subsequently processed.

The evidence gathered by the Victoria Climbié Inquiry (Laming 2003) demonstrated that practitioners from health and welfare agencies were not sharing information and that multi-agency assessment was not occurring as a matter of routine for children and families. It is essential that all local authority areas ensure that there is implementation within their area for a Common Assessment Framework to be used in the assessment of vulnerable children and young people who are in need of service (DFES 2005). For health professionals, this requires that the Common Assessment Framework will need to be reflected in the nursing assessment of some children and families.

Within the UK, the role that nurses play within the child protection process has not been evident. While key professions such as medicine and social work are prominent, other health and welfare professionals appear to serve a lesser role even when the knowledge, which individual practitioners may hold about a family may have been crucial to informing any child protection process. For example, the role of education and a child's classroom teacher has only recently been recognised as being crucial.

Other countries, such as Australia, have had mandatory reporting by all public sector professionals of child protection concerns since the 1970s (Nayda 2004). To date, this has not happened in the UK although since the Victoria Climbié case (Laming 2003) the phrase 'child protection is everybody's business' is frequently quoted within the health care setting, and the shift from the child protection process being seen as a separate procedure to one where it is part of a whole philosophy of safeguarding of children and young people has become more prolific, supported by recent legislation (Children Act 2004, *Every Child Matters* 2004).

Similar to other public sector agencies such as education, the need for nurses to be reporting their concerns about any individual child has only recently become evident. To some extent, there is resistance. Nurses, even within children's health services in the UK, have only recently had mandatory training with respect to child protection and safeguarding issues. Because child protection was seen as outside the remit of the health care setting, nurses may even say that their speciality of nursing does not relate to child protection and is the reason that they 'don't do the subject'! Nayda (2004) found evidence that nurses were not always explicit in raising their concerns about a child's welfare. Although they would pass information on to other professionals within the health care setting, this was often through more informal means and did not involve written documentation of those concerns. This was also highlighted by Laming (2003) as a shortcoming of nursing staff in the Victoria Climbié Inquiry.

The reason for this resistance to reporting of concerns about a child arises from a number of factors. Firstly, nursing staff say that they are afraid to report as this may be making a judgement of the family and that they may have read the signs wrong. Secondly the nurse's perception that she is the advocate for the family, rather than that of the child, may influence that nurse to enter into a collusive relationship with the adults in the family. This is made more difficult in that a core part of training for nurses is the concept of family-centred care and the inclusion of parents and other significant carers as partners within that process. This can challenge boundaries of professional practice with blurring of the professional relationship occurring between patient, carer and professional. This may ultimately affect the health care offered to the patient and may disrupt the routines for other patients on the ward.

Case Scenario 3

Rianne is 14 years old and was diagnosed with diabetes at 5 years. She has had an increasing number of admissions to hospital due to non-compliance with her medication. She has recently taken an overdose and tells staff that if she is sent home she will commit suicide. She does not want her mother to visit her on the ward. Rianne's mother tells her that if Rianne does not allow her to visit then she will not be able to supply her with money for her mobile telephone or for other needs while she is an inpatient. Nurses on the ward make a decision that Rianne's mother is being unreasonable with her daughter and they bring Rianne money cards for her mobile telephone and bring back treats from their holidays for her. It is 3 months into Rianne's admission that any health practitioner feels that there may be a need to make referral to other agencies or that Rianne's stay on the ward cannot continue. The child protection nurse instigated supervision sessions with the nurses involved in Rianne's care. The need to be aware of the need for professional boundaries to be reasserted was discussed. This involved exploring with nursing staff their duty of care to Rianne, to her family and to one another.

Within nurse education, and particularly disciplines that provide children's services, the concept of seeing delivery of health care as being family centred is internalised in legislative frameworks (Children Act 1989, 2004) and within nursing models for the delivery of health care to children and families (Casey 1988). Since the release of the Platt report in 1959, the need for parental involvement in the care of their children has been a priority. This is also reflected in guidance delivered to other professions such as social work (Children Act 1989, Thorburn *et al.* 1995).

Within nursing, this has led nurses to view the needs of children and the needs of parents as being one. It is often difficult to consider the child's needs as being independent from those of the parents. When there is a need to consider that the parent may not be acting in the best interest of the child or that they may have caused injury to that child, a potential situation of conflict arises in which the nurse may find it hard to comprehend that a parent has not acted within a child's best interest. In some cases, this may lead to nurses colluding with parents or attempting to minimise extent of harm suffered by the child. Lloyd and MacDonald (2000) felt that practitioners from all disciplines often have difficulty in the concept that patients and parents may give false information within the health assessment.

In the case of children who may have a complex or chronic health condition this may lead to health practitioners ignoring the risk to a child and trying to continue to work with the family within the altered parameters. This often results in the child's defined needs being determined by their medical condition rather than their status as a child with a medical condition.

Case Scenario 4

Lucy was born with cystic fibrosis. Her mother is 14 years old and the eldest of four children. Maternal grandmother appears to be carrying out the majority of both health and child care to Lucy. Maternal grandmother has mental health issues and her other children have both health and emotional needs that are to be met by her. When it becomes evident that the family are having difficulties caring for Lucy through non-attendance of appointments and non-compliance with health care, the nursing and medical team feel that it is not wise to enlist the assistance of other agencies such as social services as Lucy's care is as good as it can be given due to the social circumstances of the family. The child protection nurse discussed with practitioners the need for Lucy to be viewed as a child with a health condition rather than vice versa and also whether they considered that if Lucy did not have a chronic health problem then would parenting of Lucy meet all her needs as a child. All agreed that they did not believe that her parenting was adequate. Referral was made to other agencies to enhance support to Lucy and other members of her family. This included persuading Lucy's grandmother to seek help for her mental health.

The need to examine how the term 'partnership with parents' is defined has been a key role within child protection nursing. The difficulties described above often develop because there has been a lack of clarity from the outset of the relationship being initiated between the parent, the child and the nurse as to the expectations of the role that each is expected to carry out to meet the health needs of the child. Many parents complain that they are unclear as to their role within an acute care setting with respect to their child and may feel disempowered to carry out even simple tasks such as feeding (Callery and Smith 1991, Darbyshire 1994). This may leave nurses making subjective assessment that a parent has refused or is unable to meet the needs of their child and can lead to conflict between professionals and the family. There has often been no evidence available as to how this assessment has been made and has been based on the nurse's feelings at the time.

There may also be a need for nurses to feel that the parent is in need of protection from the professional. This may be brought about by the need to break bad news to a patient with respect to the medical condition of their child or to protect the parent from the demands that a sick child may be placing or other implications that the illness has on both the individual and the wider family group. Any negative behaviours demonstrated by the parents may be interpreted by the nurse as being normal in response to stress rather than further examination, which may indicate that the demonstrated behaviour is within the normal personality of the individual. This may lead to conflict between nurses within a ward team and from other disciplines who may be participating in the care of that family as they may well have placed different meaning to the event. The focus is then also moved away from the outcome for the child of such behaviour, and the parent is the person who receives 'care' rather than the child (Lloyd and MacDonald 2000).

Case Scenario 5

A 2-year-old child is admitted to the ward with symptoms indicating that she may have been sexually abused. Both parents tell the nurse that they do not understand how their daughter could have suffered this abuse as they have been her sole carers and would not harm her in such a way. The parents tell the nurse that she has helped them to get through the day as they know that she believes that they have not been the perpetrators of the abuse. The nurse feels that the parents are genuine in their remorse and becomes upset when the on-call doctor informs the parents that there is a need for social services and the police to be involved in the investigation. The child protection nurse explored with the nurse why she believed that the parents could not have perpetrated the abuse of their child and the process that the nurse had undertaken to reach that conclusion. The discussion questioned the judgements that health staff make of all families who present to us, the speed in which conclusion is made by the health professional and the blurring of boundaries between the health professional and the patient and/or carer. The child protection nurse questioned the nurse's perception of her role and discussed that the nurse was not responsible for investigating who had perpetrated abuse against the child. The child protection nurse discussed with the nurse why she was upset for the parents rather than for the child who has potentially been subjected to abuse.

Children with special needs/chronic illness

If the needs of children in the earlier part of the 20th century were not evident in the British society, this was even more so for the needs of disabled children and young people. What was evident, however, was that there appeared to be an incomprehension that children who may either have a disability or a chronic illness may also be suffering abuse. Watson (1989) described his horror when he first realised that a child who he had known well had been sexually abused.

It came as a shock. My own view of social reality was that handicapped children were sacrosanct, not to be touched (p. 113).

Watson states that there are six reasons as to why disabled children are at risk of suffering abuse. Firstly, there is a cultural belief that children who may be deviant from the normal child may be rejected by society. Secondly, the child may have behaviours that Watson says are abuse-provoking behaviours such as hyperactivity. Thirdly, there may be extra stresses on care givers to care for a child with a disability. Fourthly for children and young people who receive services or may who live in residential settings, there may be evidence that behaviour modification regimes may lead to abusive behaviours. Fifthly there may be also a decision made that a child with a disability may not be suitable to have health treatments that are available for a child without a disability. This may also include a disabled child not being able to access the same educational opportunity as a non-disabled child. Finally, the child's disability may place him/her at greater risk of vulnerability. For example, a child with limited verbal communication skills may be unable to tell of the abuse that is taking place.

The reaction of nurses to cases of suspected abuse of disabled children may provoke a number of responses including that as described by Watson. There may be a compromise to the care of the child as previously described in which nurses may accept parents delivering a standard of care that is lower to that of a child without a disability based on the factors as described by Watson. What has also been evident is the belief by nurses and other health disciplines that because a child has a disability it may be harder or impossible for a child to be placed with foster parents, who may need specialised skills to meet the child's needs. The result of this belief is that suspected abuse of a disabled child remains unreported (Kennedy and Wonnacott 2005).

Case Scenario 6

Liam is 8 years old. He has severe cerebral palsy and is unable to mobilise or communicate verbally. On two occasions, he has been admitted – once with a fracture to the left humerus and on another occasion with burns to his left leg. His mother says that on the first occasion, he has fallen from a pram that was parked at the top of the stairs in the family home. There was no explanation for the burn. Decision is made by the nursing and medical team that Liam's mother is under enough stress at the present time as Liam's care needs have increased recently. A referral is not made to other agencies as, in the opinion of health staff, Liam may be difficult to place in foster care. The child protection nurse explored staff the depth of questioning of parents with respect to gaining a history as to how the injuries for Liam had occurred and why staff believed that Liam's injuries should not be examined in the same manner as would occur if Liam was a child who did not have a disability. Discussion also occurred as to why assessment of the family's circumstances had not concluded that there was a greater rather than lesser reason for other agencies to be involved with the family so that the family could access more services to support their needs. Referral was made to social service team that allocated a social worker from the disability team. Liam was allocated a support worker, and monthly respite care was found for Liam.

Adult services

The organisation of health and welfare service provision is arranged according to categories such as age, gender, disability, and health condition of the service user. This leads to a philosophy of care that focuses on the needs of the individual by the practitioner. The most recent shift in the philosophy of safeguarding children and young people has forced practitioners from diverse areas of health to consider not just the needs of the patient before them but also the effects of the individual's condition and its implications for the wider family unit (Home Office 2003, Laming 2003). This has been a major shift for those practitioners who provide health services to adults. Practitioners have needed to review information sharing about their client groups. This has led to some conflict especially when disclosure of sensitive information is necessary (Murphy and Harbin 2000). Nurses working within the adult areas are being asked to share information with respect to issues such as domestic violence, mental health and drug and alcohol use. Furthermore, Section 11 of the Children Act 2004 places an onus on these practitioners to raise concerns about their patient's capacity to parent a child. Previously, risk factors for adults with respect to vulnerability have been seen as separate to the risk of other family members, especially children. This is reflected in child protection mandatory training for most health care organisations being focused on meeting the needs of health professionals who work within children's services rather than elsewhere. Furthermore, the subject of vulnerable adults is seen as separate to that of vulnerable child (Murphy and Oulder 2000).

Domestic violence, substance use and mental and physical ill health of adults

Domestic violence kills two women per week in the UK, and one in four women will be affected by this issue at some point in their lives (DH 2000b). Domestic violence and its effects on family life have been traditionally viewed as a separate factor for vulnerability, having implications only for women, within the family setting. Later research has also identified that males may also be the subject of domestic violence, and violence may also occur in same-sex relationships. Research from the late 1980s has revealed that there is a link between the profiles of adults who abuse other adults and those who perpetuate abuse against children. An extensive number of research studies carried out in Australia, Canada, America and the UK (Gardiner 1995, Brandon and Lewis 1996, Findlater and Kelly 1999, Margolin and Gordis 2000) all give similar figures stating that in households where domestic violence has been disclosed 60% of children are also suffering physical abuse and emotional abuse. Conversely, in families where child physical abuse has been identified, 60% of women are suffering domestic violence. Starke and Flitcraft (1988) felt that there was a need to emphasise that the mere act of a child witnessing domestic violence placed that child at risk of emotional harm and, therefore, should be seen as an emotionally abusive act. The definition for emotional abuse of a child has now been extended to include children who witness acts of domestic violence (DFES 2006).

Women who are suffering from domestic violence reason that their abusive partner may use physical violence towards her but does not use violence towards any children who may also be living within the family. Abrahams (1994) reported that one reason for women making such statements was that if they made frank disclosure as to the effects of the domestic abuse on family life then their children may be removed into the care system.

While DH guidance in the UK and many health trust child protection policies encourage staff to report acts of domestic violence against women who are caring for children, health staff are often reluctant to report such incidents to child protection services. Recent guidance from the Home Office (Greater Manchester Police 2006) advises that all women who are attending Accident and Emergency Departments with injuries, sustained through violence, should be risk assessed and their right to confidentiality wavered by health professionals whether or not the woman has children and if the level of further risk to either herself or to others is assessed as high.

Rivett and Kelly (2006) argue, however, that the linking of domestic violence to child protection procedures may not be the best way to help families. They argue that the all children, estimated 750,000 (DH 2002), who witness domestic violence within the UK cannot be possibly offered a service by health and welfare agencies, and by reporting all cases, professionals may actually minimise the services that can be offered to families. They state that there is a need for risk assessment to be made with respect to the whole family need and assessment made of the outcomes that the violent act may be having on the child.

Case Scenario 7

A woman attended the Accident and Emergency Department, accompanied by the police and the woman's 3-year-old daughter. She had sustained injuries to her eyes after her partner had sprayed furniture polish into her eyes. The woman had been sitting with her 3-year-old daughter on her knee earlier that evening when the injury had occurred. Her injuries were treated. No further action was taken by health staff as the police were already involved in the case. There was no attempt to examine the 3-year-old girl for injury even though she had been on her mother's knee when the injury had occurred. The child protection nurse questioned staff action as to why examination of the 3-year-old child had not occurred and why the need for the child to be also safeguarded from harm had not been considered. Staff felt that the child had only been a victim of violence given the physical proximity to her mother on that evening and that normally there was no risk to the child. The context in which the child and the mother lived was seen separately with the risk of violence being seen as a risk only to the mother.

Factors such as mental ill health, drug and alcohol use and chronic illness of a parent may have implications for children as, in the absence of other support networks within the family, the child may act as carer for the parent, so altering the parent–child relationship. Alison (2000) highlighted numerous studies undertaken internationally, which have linked parental drug and alcohol usage with child neglect. She goes on to state that there may be many reasons linking parental drug use and child abuse together including poor parenting skills, a history of abuse in the parent's own childhood and that needing to identify resources to meet the parent's drug habit distracts the parent from their role of parenting. Cleaver *et al.* (1999) concluded that drug use, mental ill health and domestic violence were often interlinked in adults and had the effect of making parents emotionally unavailable for their child. This also resulted in children not attending school or health appointments. Laybourn *et al.* (1997) looked at the perspectives of children with respect to their parents' drug use. The children described living a family life of secrets in that the drug use was a secret, which they did not speak about either with their parents or with others outside of the home environment. Minty (2005) advocates the importance of ensuring that assessment of risk to children of harm from parents with mental ill health, drug and alcohol use and from chronic physical illness needs to be assessed by the multi-agency teams, not by social workers alone. This assessment may also need to include the ability of some children to meet the needs of their parents' health status, and assessment of the needs of the adult may need to be balanced, ensuring that the needs of the child or young person are also met. The implication for the practice of health workers is that there is a need to overcome the barriers, which have often been built as a protective structure around the professional and the patient, if effective information sharing is to occur and ultimately effective support and positive outcomes can be achieved for the family.

Case Scenario 8

Francis is 30 years old and suffers from multiple sclerosis. She has four children under the age of 12 years and has been a single parent since the children's father left the family home 3 years ago. Nursing staff in the outpatient department noted that Francis always attended the hospital with all her children present and that both Francis and her children appeared to look unkempt and had poor personal hygiene. This was referred to the child protection team at the hospital as nurses questioned whether abuse of the children through neglect was occurring. When Francis was asked by the child protection nurse how her illness affected her family life, she told her that her 12-year-old Joanne was her main carer. This sometimes meant that Joanne needed to take time off school when Francis was unwell and that Joanne needed to take the other children to school and nursery everyday. Joanne was having difficulty moving her mother to help her into the bath and could only cook basic food for the family when Francis was unwell. Referral was made to the family health visitor, and the children's respective school nurses were made aware of the children's situation. A social worker for Francis was identified, and a care worker was allocated to her to help with housework and to apply for finances. All the above was documented in Francis's discharge plan at the hospital.

Conclusion

The shift of focus for health organisations from meeting the physical needs of the child within a medical-focused model of health care to that which considers health as part of the whole make up of the family has increased the role for nurses in supporting families in ensuring that children meet health outcomes. The National Service Framework for Children, Young People and Maternity Services (DFES 2004) sets out to ensure that both social and health aspects of a family life are incorporated into services offered by health and welfare services for families, with all agencies needing to be able to demonstrate by 2014 that their respective services are addressing specific outcomes for children and families. This has an impact on the present defined roles of each profession involved in safeguarding of children with boundaries of what each service from each agency is expected to provide to a family. During the past 15 years in the UK, nursing has seen a shift from nurses identifying concerns about the welfare of a child and reporting these to medical staff, who would be charged to take appropriate action on information, to nurses being accountable for reporting concerns whether or not other disciplines within the health team are in agreement. Since 2004, however, nurses also have a part to play in the assessment of need of the family and to arrange services to meet those needs as far as possible. For example, health care specialist nurses who are defined by the disease of the group of children which they care for, for example, diabetes, cystic fibrosis and cancers, may spend much of their role addressing social issues of the family so that compliance with treatment is effective. There may be also a need to offer advice on issues previously outside the traditional remit of that role such as help with benefits for the family and accessing nursery placement for either the child with the condition or for siblings.

Within health there are implications for the way that health organisations work together. There is realisation that the traditional boundaries to the provision of effective health care for families based on age of each family member, medical condition and whether the individual's health need is seen as being met within a primary, secondary or tertiary care setting are now being broken down, the emphasis being that the need to provide health care to families and the seeking of common ground for all nurses being identified. What is evident is not just the individual journey through health care but the impact of that journey for all family members.

References

Abrahams C (1994). *The Hidden Victims: Children and Domestic Violence*. London: NCH Action for Children.

Alison L (2000). What are the risks to children of parental substance misuse? In: Harbin F and Murphy M (eds), *Substance Misuse and Child Care*. Dorset: Russell House.

Brandon M and Lewis A (1996). Significant harm and children's experience of domestic violence. *Child and Family Social Work*, 1, 33–42.

Bridge Childcare Consultancy (1995). *Paul: Death Through Neglect*. London: Bridge Consultancy Services.

Caffey F (1946). Multiple fractures in the long bones of children suffering from chronic subdural haematoma. *American Journal of Roentgenology and Radium Therapy*, 56, 163–173.

Callery P and Smith L (1991). A study of role negotiation between nurses and the parents of hospitalised children. *Journal of Advance Nursing*, 16, 772–781.

Casey A (1988). A partnership with child and family. *Senior Nurse*, 8(4), 8–9.

Children Act (1989). London: HMSO.

Children Act (2004). London: HMSO.

Cleaver H, Unell I and Aldgate J (1999). *Children's Needs – Parenting Capacity: The impact of Parental Mental Illness, Problem Alcohol and Drug use and Domestic Violence on the Development of Children.* London: HMSO.

Committee of Inquiry (1974). *The Care and Supervision Provided in Relation to Maria Colwell.* London: HMSO.

Dale P (2004). 'Like a fish in a bowl': Parents' perceptions of child protection services. *Child Abuse Review*, 13, 137–157.

Darbyshire P (1994). *Living with a Sick Child in Hospital.* London: Chapman and Hall.

De Mause L (ed) (1974). *The History of Childhood.* New York: Psychohistory press.

Department for Education and Skills (DFES) (2002). The Joint Chief Inspectors' Report. London: HMSO.

Department for Education and Skills (DFES) (2004). *Every Child Matters: Change for Children.* London: HMSO.

Department for Education and Skills (DFES) (2006a). *The Common Assessment Framework for Children and Young People.* London: HMSO.

Department for Education and Skills (DFES) (2006b). *Working Together to Safeguard Children. A Guide to Safeguard and Promote the Welfare of Children.* London: HMSO.

Department of Health (DH) (1988). *Protecting Children, a Guide for Social Workers Undertaking a Comprehensive Assessment.* London: HMSO.

Department of Health (DH) (1995). *Clarification of Arrangements Between the NHS and Other Agencies.* London: HMSO.

Department of Health (DH) (1998). *Quality Protects: Transforming Children's Service.* London: HMSO.

Department of Health (DH) (1999). *Working Together to Safeguard Children. A guide to Interagency Working to Safeguard and Promote the Welfare of Children.* London: HMSO.

Department of Health (DH) (2000a). *Framework for the Assessment of Children in Need and Their Families.* London: HMSO.

Department of Health (DH) (2000b). *Domestic Violence: A Resource Manual for Health Care Professionals.* London: HMSO.

Department of Health (DH) (2001). *Learning From Bristol. The Report of the Public Inquiry into Children's Heart Surgery at Bristol Royal Infirmary from 1984 to 1995.* London: HMSO.

Department of Health (DH) (2002a). *Safeguarding Children: A Joint Chief Inspector's report on Arrangements to Safeguard Children.* London: HMSO.

Department of Health (DH) (2002b). *Women's Mental Health: Into the Mainstream. Strategic Development of Mental Health Care for Women.* London: HMSO.

Department of Health (DH) (2004). *The National Service Framework for Children, Young People and Maternity Services.* London: HMSO.

Findlater J and Kelly S (1999). Reframing child safety in Michigan: Building collaboration amongst domestic violence, family preservation and child protection services. *Child Maltreatment*, 2(2), 167–174.

Gardiner J (1995). Is the glass empty or half full? Action against domestic violence in Australia. In: Harwin N, Hague G and Malso E (eds), *The multiagency Approach to Domestic Violence: New Opportunities New Challenges?* London: Whiting and Birch.

Gibbons J, Conroy S and Bell C (1995a). *Operating the Child Protection System: A Study of Child Protection Practices in English Local Authorities*. London: HMSO.

Gibbons J, Gallagher B, Bell C and Gordon D (1995b). *Development After Physical Abuse in Early Childhood: A Follow up Study of Children on Child Protection Registers*. London: HMSO.

Greater Manchester Police (2006). *Domestic Abuse Information Sharing Protocol and Assessment Threshold*. Manchester: Greater Manchester Police.

Hallett C and Birchall E (1995). *Coordination and Child Protection*. London: HMSO.

Health Care Commission (2005). *Standards for Better Health*. London: HMSO.

Home Office (1945). *Report by Sir Robert Monkton KCMG, KCVO, MC, KC on the circumstances which led to the boarding out of Denis and Terrance O'Neill at Bank Farm, Minsterley, and the steps taken to supervise their welfare*. London: HMSO.

Home Office (2003). *Safety, and Justice: Sharing Personal Information in the Context of Domestic Violence – an Overview*. London: HMSO.

Kempe HC, Silverman FN, Steele BF, Droegemuller W and Silver HK (1962). The Battered – Child Syndrome. *Journal of the American Medical Association*, 181, 17–24.

Kennedy M and Wonnacott J (2005). Neglect of disabled children, Chapter 2. In: *Child Neglect Practical Issues for Health and Social Care*. London: Jessica Kingsley.

Laming H (2003). *The Victoria Climbié Inquiry*. London: HMSO.

Laybourn A, Brown J and Hill M (1997). *Hurting on the inside: Child Experiences of Parental Drug Misuse*. Tyne and Wear: Avebury press.

Lloyd H and Macdonald A (2000). Picking up the pieces. In: Eminson M and Postlethwaite RJ (eds), *Munchausen Syndrome by Proxy Abuse*. Oxford: Butterworth-Heinemann.

Margolin G and Gordis EB (2000). The effects of family and community violence on children. *Annual Review of Psychology*, 51, 445–479.

Minty B (2005). *The Nature of Emotional Child Neglect and Abuse*. As cited in Child Neglect. Practice issues for health and social care, Chapter 2. London: Jessica Kingsley.

Murphy M and Harbin F (2000). *Substance Misuse and Child Care*. Dorset: Russell House.

National Society for the prevention of Cruelty to Children (NSPCC) (2004). *A pocket History of the NSPCC*. London: NSPCC.

Nayda R (2004). Registered nurses' communication about child abuse. Rules, responsibilities and resistance, *Child Abuse Review*, 13, 188–199.

Parton N, Thorpe D and Wattam C (1997). *Child Protection: Risk and Moral Order*. Basingstoke: Palgrave.

Platt D (2006). Threshold decisions: How social workers prioritise referrals of child protection concern. *Child Abuse Review*, 15, 4–18.

Platt Report (1959). *The Welfare of Children in Hospital*. London: Ministry of Health.

Reder P, Duncan S and Gray M (1998). *Beyond Blame. Child Abuse Tragedies Revisited*. London: Routledge.

Rivett M and Kelly S (2006). From Awareness to Practice: Children, Domestic Violence and Child Welfare. *Child Abuse Review*, 15, 224–242.

Roper N, Logan W and Tierney A (1996). *The Roper, Logan Tierney Model of Nursing*. London: Churchill Livingstone.

Starke E and Flitcraft A (1988). Women and Children at risk: A feminist perspective on child abuse. *International Journal of Health Services*, 9(3), 97–118.

Thorburn J, Lewis A and Shemmings D (1995). *Paternalism or Partnership? Family Involvement on the Child Protection Process*. London: HMSO.

Watson G (1989). The abuse of disabled children and young people. In: Stanton Rogers W, Hevey D and Ash E (eds), *Child Abuse and Neglect, Facing the Challenge*. London: Open University.

Part 3
Advancing Nursing Roles in Children and Young People's Nursing

Introduction

Jane Hughes and Geraldine Lyte

Part 3 provides a detailed analysis of advanced practice in children's nursing. It begins with a chapter focusing on the advanced practitioner in emergency and assessment areas, giving an overview of the development of the advanced nurse practitioner and how practitioners work towards the necessary training and education for the role. Skills in acute assessment triage and clinical decision making are discussed, and two case studies are included which give a clear illustration of the advanced skills that are required in these settings.

The second chapter adds to this by giving a generic overview of the development of such roles and the advanced skills portfolio. It then includes a number of case studies of children's nurses from a wide range of specialist roles.

The third chapter focuses on the development of nursing roles and research and education in children's nursing. The concluding chapter focuses on the longer term scope of practice for children's nurses.

Chapter 10
The Advanced Practitioner in Emergency and Acute Assessment Units

Jo Bennett and Jane Hughes

Introduction: an overview

The past 50 years have witnessed a remarkable journey in a bid to raise the profile of children's nursing. The major drive behind this journey has been to change the attitude of the National Health Service (NHS) towards children. Until recently, children have been viewed as miniature adults, with very little recognition being given towards their individual- or family-specific needs. There have been several important documents that have helped to carve the pathway for where children's nursing is today, including The Welfare of Children in Hospital (1959); Fit for the Future (1976); The White Paper 'Working for Patients, Children Act' (1989); The Response to Learning from Bristol, 'Department of Health (DH)' (2001b); Department for Education and Skills (DfEs) and Department of Health (DH) (2004) and The Victoria Climbie Inquiry (2003), to name a few. The generic theme underlying each document echoes the belief that the staff caring for children view them as different from adults. They aspire to build and deliver services that have been designed and delivered for the needs of children and their families, rather than for the professional or the organisation. The idea of providing 'joined up, seamless care' and the 'provision of effective, safe care through appropriately trained and skilled staff, working in a suitable, child friendly environment' is paramount to the future development of Children's Services (NSF for Children, Chapter 2; Standard for Hospital Services 2003).

This chapter focuses in depth on the role of the experienced practitioner and the scope of advancing practice extending beyond defined nursing boundaries. Scope can simply be regarded as the activities that an individual health care practitioner is permitted to perform within a specific profession.

The chapter will provide an overview of the following:

- Role development
- Education

- Settings
- Key acute settings
- The children's advanced nurse practitioner within the acute setting – A case study
- Case study of the advanced practitioner in the emergency department (ED)

Role development

The development of specialist and advanced nursing practice is not a new notion. The ever-changing health patterns of children has resulted in a NHS that strives for the development of new practices, advanced treatments and improved technology in response to the demand and expectation of high quality, accessible health care provision. As long ago as the first half of the 20th century, American nurses with extensive expertise and experience considered themselves to be specialised practitioners. This specialisation resulted in nurses with an increased knowledge, far greater than that expected from a novice nurse (Peplau 1965). Peplau believed that these nurses should have post-graduate education and launched the first master's course in 1954. The nurse practitioner role developed as a result of innovations in response to an increasing emphasis on primary health care and a shortage of medical staff. The initial was developed in 1965 and was run by a doctor and a nurse over a 4-month period to produce nurse practitioners for children (Hamric and Taylor 1998).

Although the concept of advanced practice has been around for over half a century, the concept of advancing practice is to a certain degree still evolving. The last three decades have witnessed a major movement within British nursing that has advocated the creation of a clinical structure that will retain expertise at the bedside, advance excellence in patient care and strengthen the profile of clinical practice. The expansion of technology and the development of specialisation have created an emphasis on the importance of academic knowledge within the nursing profession. These factors have resulted in a desire among nurses to broaden their practice and stretch professional boundaries (Castledine 1991).

The development of new nursing roles has been driven by both internal and external driving forces. Historically, there has been a tendency for nurses, working in subservience to medicine, to encompass the tasks assigned to them by their medical colleagues. However, recent acceleration appears to have been driven in response to the Calman report and the initial acknowledgement of the reduction in the hours worked by junior doctors (Hooker 1991, NHS Management Executive 1991, DH 1993). More recently, 'The Working Time Directive' for junior doctors in training continues to be a major catalyst for reviewing the way that the NHS currently delivers health care in children's services [Working Time (Amendment) Regulations 2003] (see also Fig. 11.1). As a response to these changes, the government, as part of its modernisation agenda in the NHS, grasped the opportunity to improve standards through more innovative ways of working and a changing skill mix.

Like many specialities, the concept of the children's advanced nurse practitioner is at last rapidly emerging. Until recent years, the issue of 'paediatric specialisation' for the nurse practitioner has been a complex issue (see Chapter 11). While it has long been recognised that children are a specialised group with special concerns, it has only been in recent years that there has been universal acceptance that children are a legitimate population. The children's nurse is a registered nurse with a specific body of knowledge and family-centred skills, caring for specific age groups whose needs are markedly different from those of adults. This depth and breadth of knowledge encompasses the complete physiological, psychological, spiritual, cultural and environmental needs of the infant, child and adolescent and their families (RCN 2003b). Nursing services for this population group form the basis of essential child health services. However, the development of a stronger children's nursing profile is necessary. This will make better use of already appropriate and highly qualified, experienced and skilled children's nurses and will help to raise the profile of children's nursing. The development of advanced children's roles will enable nurses to meet the complex and unique needs of children, adolescents and their families requiring health care in hospital and in the community. For further examples, see Chapter 11.

The ultimate aim of the children's advanced nurse practitioner must be to provide a holistic and comprehensive service adopting a family-centred approach, while providing continuity of care and advancing nursing practice. In terms of clinical expertise, a practitioner at this level would be accomplished in all domains of nursing care and would possess the skills of advanced health assessment (AHA), diagnosis, requesting and interpreting investigations, prescribing and evaluating care, to name a few (Benner 1984). The role will encompass five areas of competence – clinical, research, teaching, consultation and leadership outlined by Castledine (1991) and eight core competencies defined by Hamric (1989) – expert clinical practice; expert guidance and coaching of patients, families and other care providers; consultation; research skills; clinical and professional leadership; collaboration; change agent skills and ethical decision-making skills. These competencies mark advanced practice regardless of the role, function or setting and have been repeatedly identified as essential Advanced Nurse Practitioner (ANP) features that are learned by all ANPs, who then apply them to specific patient populations and settings (Hamric 1996).

The role of the children's ANP is wide and varied but would invariably strive to improve the quality of care experienced by children and their families and perhaps in addressing some of the issues raised in the National Service Framework (DH 2004) and the Health Care Commission report (2007). The key to achieving this is in developing a culture, which will facilitate staff empowerment and nursing practice development. The development of the role is an exciting venture. By being proactive, the ANP can develop their role in all aspects of AHA and in decision-making skills while delivering holistic care. The role has a clear focus on nursing and endeavours to meet the needs of children and families within the climate of today's health care. The commitment to family-centred care, education and health promotion will help to distinguish the ANP role from a medical role. Autonomy, possession of highly developed clinical skills, knowledge and an effective communicator are all essential competencies within such an advanced role. The ability to make decisions and network across boundaries play an important part of the ANP role. The role of the children's advanced nurse practitioner must be viewed as a holistic professional concept of nursing expertise reflecting the art and science of nursing care. In particular, the role of advanced practice has a much broader consequence for the future in terms of achieving targets set out by the Department of Health (DH) and the government.

In essence, the role of the ANP, and the ideology behind the clinical structure, enables children's nurses to fulfil professional and organisational demands while exhibiting their excellence in knowledge, skill and practice and while providing a service that benefits the child and family, the organisation and the practitioner.

Education for the role

The role of the children's advanced nurse practitioner supports the Royal College of Nursing definition of nursing (2003) that recognises that while nursing is the 'totality', the nursing role itself encompasses great diversity and recognises that some parts of the definition are shared with other health care professionals. However, a major concern of the Nursing and Midwifery Council (NMC), the public and many other nurses, midwives and other health care professionals has been the various different job titles given to describe experienced practitioners, which do not explicitly explain the level qualification, knowledge and competence that the practitioner has attained.

A children's advanced nurse practitioner is a children's nurse who would normally hold a master's degree in advanced nursing education, is certified as a Registered Children's Nurse and has received additional training to provide a wide range of skill, expertise and a broad range of health care services for patients. They may work within the primary, secondary, tertiary or private sector.

Following consultation on a 'Framework for the standard for post-registration nursing' (2005), a revised definition for advanced practitioners was proposed: 'Advanced nurse practitioners are highly experienced, knowledgeable and educated members of the care team who are able to diagnose and treat your health care needs or refer you to an appropriate specialist if needed'. However, the NMC recognises that while definitions are helpful, they can also have their limitations, and therefore it was decided that it would be more helpful to expand the definition to provide a more detailed overview about what patients, carers and other health care professionals can expect of an advanced nurse practitioner. A further explanation describing advanced nurse practitioners as highly skilled nurses, who are only permitted to call themselves by this title, will be protected by a registered qualification in the council's register, once they have achieved the competencies set out by the NMC that entitles the practitioner to practice in areas beyond the scope of the registered nurse:

- Carry out physical examinations.
- Use their expert knowledge and clinical judgement to decide whether to refer patients for investigations (e.g. imaging and blood investigations) and to diagnose.
- Decide on and carry out treatment, including prescription of medicines, or refer patient to an appropriate specialist.
- Use their extensive practice experience to plan and provide skilled and competent care to meet patients health and social care needs, involving other members of the health care team as appropriate.
- Ensure the provision of continuity of care team as appropriate.
- Ensure the provision of continuity of care including follow-up visits.
- Assess and evaluate, with patients, the effectiveness of the treatment and care provided and make changes as needed.
- Work independently, although often as part of a health care team that they will lead.
- As a leader of the team, make sure that each patient's treatment and care is based on best practice.

A key government policy of relevance to nurse practitioners was the expansion of nurse prescribing in May 2006. Nurses are now able to prescribe every drug on the National Formulary (with the exception of some controlled drugs), provided they do so within their own field of competence. This role further enhances the development of autonomous and seamless care.

Key acute care settings

Children's Assessment Units

The practice of caring for children when they are ill but do not require hospitalisation is termed paediatric ambulatory care. Ambulatory care is the provision of health services on a day service basis. The provision of ambulatory care is growing in paediatrics. Minimisation to the disruption of the lives of children and their families due to illness and hospitalisation has been high on the agenda for consumer groups and service providers for the past two decades. Nationally, we are seeing a trend towards 'one-shop' medicine, driven by high public expectation.

Ambulatory care is a facility that provides medical care including diagnosis, investigation, observation, treatment and evaluation with follow-up care. This initiative has resulted in response to a number of initiatives set out by the (DH). Firstly, children should only be admitted to hospital if the care that they require cannot equally be provided at home (Audit Commission 1993), and secondly, children should be cared for by children's nurses within facilities dedicated to the care of children (DH 1991). It is a concept driven by the NHS modernisation agenda to provide facilities and services that are convenient to the child and the family. The Royal College of Paediatrics and Child Health (RCPCH) (2003) issued a statement on ambulatory paediatrics, 'to provide care without hospital admission whenever possible and when admission is needed, to reduce it's duration to a minimum'. Ambulatory paediatrics describes care that does not require admission to hospital, apart from a few hours when the child is assessed, examined, a plan of care devised and treatment prescribed if necessary. The primary aim is to avoid inappropriate hospitalisation of children and thereby reduce the number of children admitted for inpatient care.

Ambulatory care has become an increasing emphasis within paediatrics in meeting the target to reduce at least 25% of acute hospital inpatient bed days occupied by children aged 0–15 years (HPSS Management Plan 1999/2000 to 2001/2002). Such a service requires considerable flexibility that takes into account of the needs of parents and children and the geographic and demographic characteristics of the population served (CREST 2001). More recently, national documents have reinforced the need to make changes to deliver high quality care (DH 2003a, 2007).

For such a service to flourish and function effectively, the development of a paediatric community or home care team should be considered. Children should only be hospitalised if clinically appropriate and if deemed necessary, and the duration should be kept as brief as possible with community-based services supporting the discharge of children to their own home as soon as safe to do so.

The Children's Assessment Unit (CAU) model of care is based on the philosophy that 'children should not be admitted to hospital unless absolutely necessary'. The main purpose of the CAU is to prevent inappropriate children being admitted to hospital for inpatient care. Assessment units provide an alternative to traditional hospital admission for children who need a period of short-term assessment or observation. For many children and their carers, this is a more appropriate service than admission to the main inpatient service. A core philosophy of the service should be that in many instances, nursing care of children is best delivered in their own homes using a family-centred approach. Research demonstrates that when a child is cared for in their own home, the family adjust more quickly and that home care supported with appropriate staff provides more personal care that is individualised to the family lifestyle and also a more effective use of resources. The added support from a children's home care team can facilitate early discharge whereby children who may have been previously admitted to hospital can be discharged home with support from the team. The introduction of the CAU has confirmed that effective operation can provide safe and valued service to local children, carers and general practitioners. Effective operation relies on close contact with local primary care teams, effective integrative nursing and medical staff and a community children's service (CREST 2001). The CAU will continue to expand, with acute children's hospital services providing diagnostic services on an outpatient basis.

General practitioners, medical staff in the A&E department who require further assessment, observation or investigation, Health Visitors, Midwives, School Health Advisors and other members of the multidisciplinary team, generally make referrals to the CAU. Attendance will also include those children who require a follow-up review after discharge by the paediatric team rather than within primary care. This may include children who require daily review and/or intravenous antibiotics.

Telephone communication followed by a written referral letter should take place between all refers and the staff in the Unit prior to referral, allowing further exchange of information or advice to be given.

CAU support the Accident & Emergency (A&E) service by allowing children to be transferred out of the A&E department to a dedicated facility with staff who can provide assessment and acute treatment. Having dedicated children's trained staff allows these specialised nursing and medical staff to spend more time with the children and carers to explain their illnesses and the treatment to be given, which may prevent the need for an overnight stay in hospital, improves the quality of care offered to children and their carers and prevents readmission. Equally, transferring children out of A&E will help move the patients through the A&E department more quickly, will help to reduce delayed waiting times and prevent 4-hour breaches, one of the government's performance targets. Paediatric care has changed significantly in recent years and recognises a major shift of care closer to home. Children are admitted for shorter inpatient stays, and those requiring longer stays are more likely to require high dependency care. More children are surviving with chronic long-term conditions. Where possible, children should be cared for with nursing support at home.

The maximum duration of observation varies between units and depends on the time of day and the hours of operation of the unit. In which time a decision should have been made whether the child needs admission to hospital or can be safely discharged home into the community with or without follow-up support. Discharge is supported by written advice, a direct telephone number to the unit and a 24-hour open access back to the unit whereby carers can return with their child should they have any concerns regarding their child's condition.

All assessment units operate on an individual basis. Services need to be designed to meet local needs and characteristics. However, they must be managed as an integral part of a comprehensive inpatient acute paediatric service with effective systems in place to ensure consistency and continuity of quality care between the departments, including appropriately qualified, experienced and skilled nursing, medical and clerical staff and appropriate equipment.

In view of the trends of the past decade, children's services continue to strive to provide a higher basic standard of emergency care, delivered by appropriately trained staff. Changes in health care delivery make it increasingly likely that children accessing ambulatory care will receive their health assessment and management from nurses rather than junior doctors. Alterations in the working hours of junior doctors and in the training and service developments within the NHS, in line with governmental directives, have resulted in nurses who care for children exploring new ways of working. The role of a advanced paediatric nurse practitioner (APNP) represents a convergence of three national policy streams including modernisation, advanced nursing care for infants, children and young people and also signifies a shift from the traditional model of care service delivery and promotes that all children are an important strand of the larger acute care system. The role of the APNP within the acute setting is to assess, diagnose and manage a wide variety of conditions that present to the CAU. The role also promotes health promotion and disease protection and allows child and parental support, developmental advice, screening and education.

Children's emergency department

As indicated earlier, children constitute a considerable percentage of attendees in EDs, around 28% of all attendees per year (Health Care Commission 2007), the equivalent of 2.9 million children.

There have been moves over recent years in improving specific provision for children attending ED in the UK following recommendations in the children's NSF (DH 2004). Child friendly facilities have been recognised as being helpful for children when attending departments, such as play areas, children's cubicles and children's resuscitation areas. However, recent reports have highlighted the need for appropriate resources and equipment to be available for children to be cared for quickly and appropriately (RCPCH 2007).

In addition, the report 'Improving Services for Children in Hospital' (Health Care Commission 2007) highlights the key areas where children's services are not meeting children's needs such as pain and resuscitation facilities, communication and child protection, together with the availability of children's trained staff in child-specific areas. This is a particular problem in EDs that do not have separate designated children's areas as indicated in Health Care Commission that 28% of acute trust were weak in this area. In these situations, children are frequently cared for by nursing and medical staff who do not have a specialism in children's needs (Partridge 2001). Partridge (2001) also indicates that issues concerning the sharing of waiting rooms with adults can expose children to unnecessary hostile sight and sounds.

Other issues of the employment of child branch–trained staff in a general ED exist, where the nurse trained from another branch does not hold a qualification equivalent to the child branch–trained staff; the NMC placed restrictions, following the Project 2000 changes to pre-registration training (UKCC 1997), that only a child branch–trained nurse can work autonomously in the department. The most recent report – Emergency services 2007 – indicated that these issues do need to be addressed and that there should be child friendly facilities and appropriately trained staff and importantly at least one RN child-trained nurse per shift.

Separate designated children's EDs are developing across the country (38% of trusts were providing child only care; Health Care Commission 2007), and these offer facilities that are appropriate to children, play areas and other aspects of child friendly environment. Although units do not always open for the 24 hour period, many units open in response to peak demand i.e. 9am–10pm. Perhaps more importantly, it is possible to have a service that is delivered by nursing and medical staff who have specialist training and skills to support and care for children and young people. It also allows for career progression in the speciality, that is, the emergency Nurse practitioner (ENP) in children's ED.

Some children's EDs offer telephone advice to the local community, and as in the later, many departments use national or local algorithms or care pathways to ensure safe and best practice, which may base on nurse-led consultations. Recent recommendations indicate that the ED should have nursing and medical staff with expertise on all levels for looking after children, including a lead nurse and consultant for children (RCPCH 2007).

Walk in centres

NHS walk-in centres have been established as part of the government's commitment to modernise the NHS (NHS Modernisation Agency 2003). One of the main aims was to reduce demand on NHS providers, particularly, general practitioners and EDs (Harraks *et al.* 2002). The provision of walk-in centres provides an easy access stream for patients who do not necessarily require emergency care and who could be effectively treated within the primary care remit. This can greatly reduce the demand on overstretched A&E departments. Depending on the location of the walk-in centre, patients may be streamed from triage at the ED to the primary care or walk-in centre as appropriate. Walk-in centres may be located in areas of high need where local general practitioner's bases are oversubscribed or close to other health centres. Provision for children and young people within the walk-in centre may not necessarily be given by staff specifically trained in the assessment of children, although nursing staff may have appropriate experience.

Implementation of the role within the acute setting: a case study

This section provides a descriptive account of a child who was presented to hospital in need of acute medical care. Consultation process, AHA, plan of care and the key issues that were addressed to ensure that non-medical prescribing was safely and effectively implemented are discussed. To maintain anonymity and confidentiality, the child will be referred to as Jack. It is written from the perspective of a children's advanced nurse practitioner. Reflection is an essential tool utilised to support evidence-based care delivery while supporting the analytical rational for safe, effective care.

The consultation

Jack aged 3 years presented to the CAU accompanied by his parents with a history of 'breathing difficulties'. The role of the children's ANP was to immediately assess Jacks clinical needs. The acquisition of AHA skills and non-medical prescribing enable the ANP to be autonomous in practice and to exercise clinical judgement while delivering holistic care (Bear, 1995, Howard, 1997, Amitage, 1999, Kennedy Report, 2001, NSF 2003).

Model of assessment

To structure the consultation, it was necessary to utilise a model of assessment. Models of assessment support practice by building a structural framework around which effective practice can be built (Bates 2004). The SOAPIE model is just one example of model of assessment that can be utilised (Cox 2004). Although a more clinical method of assessment, its principles support the process of care that needs to be provided, and its structure is extremely coherent and simplistic to follow.

SOAPIE is defined as the systematic collection of 'subjective' (stated by the child/parents) and 'objective' data (observed by the health professional during the physical assessment). These elements form the database of the 'assessment'. Information is gathered from the perspective of both the child/parent and the practitioner. This integration promotes shared decision making and understanding. Once the data have been gathered and interpreted, a judgement regarding the child's health state can be made followed by the development of an individualised plan of care. Implementation and evaluation of the prescribed care follow (Cox 2004). The SOAPIE framework functions as a safety network by promoting a safe, holistic and effective consultation style, necessary for AHA and safe prescribing.

Communication

Good communication skills on part of the practitioner affect the outcome of any consultation (Silverman *et al.* 1998). Maguire and Pitceathly (2002), suggesting that practitioners with good communication skills identify patient(s)/carer(s) problems more accurately resulting in greater patient/carer satisfaction. Consequently, at the end of the consultation, the patient(s)/carer(s) have a better understanding of their problem(s), proposed investigations and treatment options; adherence to treatment is increased; lifestyle changes, distresses and anxieties are lessened; and patient(s)/carer(s) have an increased well-being and satisfaction with the practitioner.

For these reasons, it is important to collaborate with the child and the parents. Role clarity and the role of the consultation process will help to establish a good rapport (Bates 2004). Even though it is not possible to erase all apprehensions, the establishment of a trusting relationship impacts considerably on the outcome of the consultation and helps to make a more positive experience. Parents contribute greatly to the care and well-being of their child and are the primary source of information about their child (Castledine 1995). Encouraging the parents to tell their story is central to the consultation.

The consultation requires an environment supporting privacy and confidentiality (Silverman *et al.* 1998). A private treatment room with child friendly decor will help to reduce any apprehension associated with the consultation. A strategy utilising a non-threatening, open manner with broad questioning, active listening and appropriate use of eye contact and body language will encourage parental participation (While 2002).

As a toddler, Jack had not yet acquired the ability to effectively communicate verbally. He had the beginnings of memory and make-believe, but was unable to understand abstractions. Perceptions of threat were amplified by inaccurate understanding and limited knowledge of the situation. Communication therefore required the use of short, concrete terms. Explanations required repeating, and parental participation was encouraged (Bates 2004).

Consent

The expectations of the courts and professional bodies regarding consent are demanding. The NMC (2008) clearly states that as a registered professional it is necessary to obtain consent before giving or engaging in any treatment. To be valid, consent must be a informed one (Beckworth and Franklin 2007). It is therefore necessary to fully inform the child's parents regarding the consultation process, including any subsequent plan of care and treatment prescribed.

Consent for treatment can be given for a child only by a person with parental responsibility for that child. This covers all rights, duties and powers that a parent has over a child, including the right to consent for treatment (Children Act 1989). The courts can, however, overrule the wishes of a parent if it is believed to be in the best interests of the child (Children Act 1989). Children under the age of 16 years can give consent if it can be proven that they have a competent level of understanding. In Scotland, this is laid down in statute law (Children Act 1989). In England and Wales, it is expressed as the Fraser ruling (Fraser 1985).

Subjective assessment

A focused history of the child's recent health, activity and previous illness should be obtained from the parents. 'Jack had been well. However, overnight he had developed a dry non-productive cough and wheeze, and now appeared to be using his chest muscles to breathe. He was finding hard to talk, refused breakfast and had only taken sips of fluid from his beaker. He had had two small mucous vomits whilst coughing during the night. Parents had changed several wet nappies. There was no history of any pyrexia or rash'. Direct inquiry identified that Jack's parents were confident that he had not inhaled a foreign body (FB).

Jack had attended the CAU on five previous occasions with difficulty in breathing, nocturnal cough and wheeze. He had no known allergies and had not taking any prescribed, over-the-counter or herbal medicines. His immunisation status was up to date. There was a strong maternal and paternal family history of asthma. There were no siblings, no pets and no smokers in the family. Birth history was uneventful, having a normal vaginal delivery, birth weight 3.5 kg.

Initial evaluation of this subjective data suggested that Jack was suffering from a degree of respiratory distress. The history was not suggestive of a FB inhalation, a potential differential diagnosis as there was no evidence of an audible inspiratory stridor (a significant symptom of FB). This would be confirmed during the objective assessment.

Objective assessment

A rapid physical examination of vital function was made (airway, breathing, circulation and disability) [Advanced Paediatric Life Support (APLS) 2005].

Airway assessment

Patency of airway was assessed by the look–listen–feel method (APLS 2005). There was no visible evidence of FB inside Jack's mouth. Jack was crying and an audible expiratory wheez/e indicated that he had a patent airway and was breathing spontaneously. It was important to explain to Jack's parents that it was important to keep Jack as calm as possible to reduce his anxiety. Jack remained seated with his mother in the position that he had adopted – sitting forward with his neck extended – a recognised tripod position that provides maximum comfort and security while maintaining the airway and promoting expansion of lungs (APLS 2005).

Breathing assessment

A patent airway does not ensure adequate ventilation (APLS 2005). Breathing requires an intact respiratory centre and adequate pulmonary function with coordinated movement of the diaphragm and chest wall (APLS 2005). The pattern of respiratory illness in children is different from that in adults. These variations result from several important anatomic and physiologic differences. Children are susceptible to infection with many organisms to which adults have acquired immunity. The upper and lower airways in children are smaller and more easily obstructed by muscle swelling, secretions and FB. The thoracic cage is more compliant when there is airway obstruction and increased inspiratory effort results in marked chest wall recession and a reduction in the efficiency of breathing. Respiratory muscle fatigue can develop rapidly and result in respiratory failure and apnoea (APLS 2005).

Jack had an increased respiratory rate of 60 beats per minute (bpm) (normal 25 bpm) (APLS 2005). Tachypnoea is often the first manifestation of respiratory distress in an attempt to maintain a normal pH by increasing minute ventilation. He had a dry intermittent non-productive cough and was making an audible grunting noise, a mechanism produced by premature epiglottic closure accompanied by late expiratory contraction of the diaphragm in an attempt to increase airway pressure, thereby preserving or increasing functional residual capacity (APLS 2005). This increased work in breathing may result in nasal flaring. It is important to observe for bilateral chest movement and to observe for any abdominal excursion or subcostal/intercostal recession. Recession is easily visible in children due to high compliance of the chest wall and diaphragm and confirms an increased effort in breathing, which is an inefficient form of ventilation. Tidal volume is reduced and fatigue likely to develop in a relatively short period of time. As work of breathing increases, a greater proportion of the cardiac output must be delivered to the respiratory muscles, which in turn produces more carbon dioxide. The presence of head bobbing with each breath suggested the use of the sternomastoid muscle due to increased respiratory effort. The trachea was central, non-deviated. Auscultation of the chest revealed bilateral reduced air entry, and the presence of an expiratory wheeze suggested narrowing of the lower airways. This ruled out pneumothorax as a potential differential diagnosis but suggested asthma. There was no evidence of an inspiratory stridor. This supported the initial theory that Jack's respiratory distress had not resulted from inhalation of a FB. It was possible to rule out acute laryngotracheobronchitis (croup) due to the absence of inspiratory stridor and 'bark like cough'. Jack's age ruled out bronchiolitis (National Respiratory Training Centre 2006).

Circulatory/disability assessment

The effects of inadequate respiration can be observed by direct observation of heart rate, skin colour and mental status. Progressive respiratory distress will eventually result in hypoxia, hypercapnia and acidosis, followed by decreased muscular tone and reduced level of consciousness (Tortora and Grabowski 2000). Jack's capillary refill was less than 2 seconds, a normal response. This ruled out any circulatory insufficiency/signs of dehydration as a differential diagnosis (APLS 2005). Heart rate was 168 bpm (norm range 80–180 bpm) (APLS 2005). Children will initially demonstrate tachycardia in an attempt to maintain adequate tissue oxygenation preventing hypoxia and hypercapnia, which will result in bradycardia and acidosis. The development of bradycardia in a child with respiratory distress is ominous, usually indicating that cardiopulmonary arrest is imminent (APLS 2005).

Jack's skin was of a sallow colour and cool to touch. His temperature was 36.2°C (norm 37.2°C) (APLS 2005). The absence of pyrexia ruled out pneumonia as a differential diagnosis. The skin over his trunk and extremities was mottled, resulting from hypoxemia. His lips were pale and lightly cyanosed. Oxygen saturations were 92% in air (below 94% unacceptable) (APLS 2005) He was becoming increasingly agitated.

Diagnosis

Traditionally, diagnosis has been seen as the prerogative of the medical practitioner, with nurse involvement being informal and often unacknowledged (Baird 2000, 2001). However, the Review of The Prescribing, Supply and Administration of Medicines (Crown II) (DH 1999) stated that part of the role of the independent prescriber is to establish diagnosis and/or a management plan, suggesting that nurse involvement in diagnosis is now formally acknowledged.

In reaching a diagnosis, the practitioner goes through several stages of data collection and critical analysis (Tate, 2003, Bates 2004). This process of clinical reasoning takes place in the clinician's mind and will often appear inaccessible to the novice practitioner (Bates 2004). The critical process involves identifying abnormal data from the subjective history, identifying abnormal signs and symptoms during the physical examination and localising the findings anatomically followed by interpretation of the findings in terms of the probable diagnosis. Drawing on previous knowledge and experience about the patterns of abnormalities and disease enables the practitioner to select the most specific and critical findings to support any potential differential diagnosis. This allows the practitioner to eliminate the competing possibilities and select the most likely diagnosis. It is not always possible to reach a definite diagnosis. This uncertainty can often be difficult to tolerate and is something that nurse prescribers (NP) need to manage as they accept responsibility for their own prescribing decisions (Luker *et al.* 1998).

From the presenting history and clinical findings, a diagnosis of an acute moderate exacerbation of asthma was made. Asthma is now the commonest reason for admission of children to hospital in the UK [British Thoracic Society (BTS)/Scottish Intercollegiate Guidelines Network (SIGN)2004]. It is a chronic disease of the respiratory system characterised by a recurrent, reversible bronchoconstriction of the airways (Asthma UK 2003, 2007a, b). The patient typically presents with cough, wheeze and breathing difficulty. These symptoms were clearly characterised by Jack's history/presentation.

Evidence-based practice

Evidence-based clinical practice is an approach to decision making through consideration and application of the best evidence available when deciding how to treat an individual patient, groups of patients or populations (National Institute for Clinical Excellence 2002). It is the process of systematically reviewing, appraising and using clinical research findings to aid the delivery of optimum clinical care to patients (Rosenberg and Donaldson 1995). Examples include National Institute for Clinical Excellence (NICE) guidelines for feverish illness, head injury and urine infection together with other sources of evidence such as the Best Bets and Clinical Evidence. The BTS/SIGN (2004) has standardised asthma care by defining a clinical management pathway based on published research evidence. This pathway provides a framework for standardised asthma treatment. The aim of asthma treatment is to minimise or eliminate symptoms, improve lung function and to enable patients to control their asthma with minimal treatment/side effects (BTS/SIGN 2003). Accepted good asthma care is that patients with asthma should have their asthma medication requirements reviewed regularly, and reduced to the minimum needed to control their symptoms (BTS/SIGN 2004). Short-acting bronchodilators are used for the symptomatic relief only on symptoms of wheeze, cough and breathlessness. In children under 5 years of age, with acute mild to moderate asthma, initial treatment should be with a beta2 agonist through a pressurised metered dose inhaler (pMDI) and a spacer device with close fitting mask (BTS/SIGN 2004, British National Formulary for Children (BNFC) 2006a, p. 163). Salbutamol, 100μg (1 puff), every 15–30 seconds, up to a maximum of 1000μg (10 puffs), should be prescribed and repeated after 20–30 minutes if necessary. The aim is to maintain oxygen saturations above 94%. If the child responds to treatment, then beta2 agonists should be continued 1–4 hourly as required depending on the response (BTS/SIGN 2004).

A pMDI and a spacer are the preferred option of delivery, however, in children who have not improved after receiving this method of treatment – nebulised medication, either 2.5mg nebulised salbutamol or 5mg terbutaline with oxygen, should be prescribed and repeated every 20–30 minutes according to the response (i.e. when oxygen saturations remain less than 92% in air despite medication, the child remains too breathless to talk or eat and heart rate continues 130bpm with use of accessory muscles) (BTS/SIGN 2004).

A nebulised solution converts the drug into an aerosol for inhalation and is used to administer higher doses of drug to the airways than with standard inhalers (BNFC 2006a). If there is a poor response, 0.25μg nebulised ipratropium bromide should be prescribed (BTS/SIGN 2004). Response to treatment should include auscultation of the chest 20–30 minutes following administration of the beta2 agonist to assess respiratory effort, efficacy and effect in response to treatment [assess air entry and breathe sounds and wheeze may become biphasic or less apparent with increasing airways obstruction (are they bilateral and equal)]. A silent chest is a poor sign. Respiratory rate, heart rate and oxygen saturation should be recorded every 1–4 hourly (increasing tachycardia suggests deterioration of asthma; a bradycardia in life-threatening asthma is a pre-terminal event) (BTS/SIGN 2004).

A dose of soluble oral 20mg prednisolone should be considered.

Plan of care

Non-medical prescribing has expanded the roles, responsibilities and relationship boundaries of many professionals allied to medicine, including advanced nurse practitioners. Acknowledgement of this enhanced knowledge and skill has offered the opportunity for non-medical practitioners to achieve their full potential, while supporting the demands of society for a more streamlined, accessible and flexible service, which provides high quality care and roles that extend beyond traditional boundaries (DH 2000b, 2001a, 2002a). As a nurse practitioner, it is important to acknowledge and reserve the decision to prescribe only for those situations where it is genuinely required. The decision to prescribe must be fully justified and influenced by previous knowledge and experience and in response to the child's condition and clinical presentation.

As a non-medical prescriber, the aim of treatment is to achieve maximum control of symptoms with the minimum amount of therapy and to prevent any further deterioration in the child's symptoms. Untreated, the risk of deterioration in condition could result in the development of a life-threatening situation. Salbutamol, a beta2 agonist, using a pMDI with spacer device and mask, 100 µg (1 puff) every 15–30 seconds, up to a maximum of 1000 µg (10 puffs) to be repeated after 20–30 minutes if necessary, was prescribed. For a prescribing practitioner, previous knowledge and experience of asthma and the effect of the salbutamol supports the decision and confidence to prescribe. The administration of salbutamol using a pMDI with spacer device and mask is relatively safe and effective in the treatment of asthma in children (BNFC 2006a). It is advocated for the treatment of asthma in children by the British National Formulary for Children (BNFC) (2006) and by the BTS/SIGN (2004). A dose of soluble oral 20 mg prednisolone was prescribed.

Jack's parents were informed of the plan of care and the necessity to evaluate any response to treatment 20–30 minutes post-administration of the inhaler. If the response is poor, it would be necessary to re-administer the dose. If there was continued poor response, it would be necessary to administer salbutamol through a nebuliser.

Evaluation of care

Jack did not respond well to the salbutamol administered through the spacer (oxygen saturation remained 92% or less and heart rate 150 bpm). There was very little improvement in his respiratory effort. Salbutamol, 2.5 mg, through the nebuliser was subsequently prescribed with good effect. Jack's parents were prepared and welcomed the change in treatment. Jack required admission overnight but was discharged 48 hours later when stable on 4 hourly inhaled treatment. On discharge, salbutamol through a pMDI and spacer device with mask, one to two puff (100–200 µg) , was to be administered up to four times daily (for occasional use only). Parent inhaler technique should be demonstrated and assessed as competent before discharge. Oral prednisolone was prescribed for a total of 3 days. Jack's parents were counselled regarding the potential addition of inhaled corticosteroids to treatment following any further exacerbations of asthma or if he required the use of salbutamol three times a week or more; if he was symptomatic three times a week or more; or if he was waking one night a week. A written clinical management plan (CMP) was made for Jack's asthma care including the process to follow if the prescribed medication did not relieve his symptoms – the introduction of inhaled corticosteroids. A 48-hour open access to the CAU was given to Jack's parents on discharge in case of deterioration of Jack's condition. A follow-up appointment should be arranged before discharge in line with local policy. Members of the primary health care team should be informed of the admission, treatment prescribed and subsequent follow-up care and CMP.

Concordance

Concordance plays an important part in the effectiveness of treatment and follow-up care. The notion of concordance is relatively new and replaces that of compliance (Cox 2004). Concordance is seen as an agreement or partnership between practitioner and patient/carer where an agreement is made to work together for the benefit of the patient and is defined as the informed partnership agreement that is negotiated between the prescriber and the patient (and/or carer in the field of Paediatrics) (Beckworth and Franklin 2007, p. xxiv). Not all patients/carers want to play a dominant role in medical care and prefer to play a passive entity whereby they are told what they must do (Cox 2004). However, all parents must be given information about their child's condition and treatment options. This will encourage parental participation by informing and empowering them with the necessary information to engage in their child's care. Jack's parents were open to suggestion and clearly valued the advice and support offered to them as a family.

The Advanced Nurse Practitioner in the emergency department: children's ENP

This section provides an account of a child with a minor injury, who is assessed by an experienced ENP in a children's ED.

Harry, a 3-year-old child, presented to the A&E department with his grandparents complaining of leg pain. After being shown initially to the paediatric waiting area, he was called to the consulting area with his family by the children's ENP. The ENP introduced herself to the family explaining her role. When treating children, it is important that the practitioner has the ability to converse with the accompanying adult and the child; experience and skills acquired from working in this field would be evident and hopefully reflected in the child and family's reaction during the assessment process (see Spotting the Sick Child DH 2004).

Harry had attended the department with two family members, and on further questioning, it was established that the maternal grandparents had bought Harry to the ED as they had been unable to contact his mother. The DH (2001a) current legislation states that consent to treatment can only be given by a parent, legal guardian or local authority if the child is in care. Although Harry's parent had not given formal consent at this point, the children's ENP decided to treat Harry as she felt that it was in his best interests and grandparents had been given responsibility for his care and had brought him to the ED. Harry's mother would be contacted before discharge and all information would be relayed to her.

Taking a comprehensive history is an extremely important part of evaluating an injury, doing so accurately gives vital cues to diagnosis. Oliver (1996) describes how history-taking should form the main part of the paediatric examination and can be an excellent opportunity to establish rapport with both child and family. While the history was taken, Harry sat on his grandfather's knee, and the children's ENP tried to include Harry in the conversation as much as possible, lowering herself to his level and listening carefully when he spoke, to try to establish all the necessary information with his grandparents assessing. Taking a history should establish the presenting complaint, when, where, why, how and what happened next, also noting patient's description of immediate symptoms after the injury (Guly 1996). The history would also include drug allergies, past medical history, regular medication and social history.

From the history, it was established that Harry had been at his grandparents' home and, 2 hours before the injury, was given a ride on the back of his 6-year-old brother and had fallen to the floor, a distance of approximately 1 foot, and he cried immediately and refused to walk. Harry had his usual sleep although remained upset before he went to sleep. When he awoke, he again refused to walk and therefore grandparents brought him to theED.

A systematic physical examination helps to clarify diagnosis and management options and ensures that associated injuries are not overlooked. Gray-Seiler (2002) describes examination as something that should be simple, systematic, comprehensive and well practised. In this instance, the approach utilised was the look–feel–move approach (Wardrope and English 1998), which the children's ENP had become practised in her clinical training. The approach to the examination, particularly in this age group, must be opportunistic and may not follow the usual order, as children do not necessarily co-operate as expected (Oliver 1996).

Harry was initially being carried; however, the ENP asked if he could be put down to establish if he could bear weight – the ability to take four steps or two transfers is defined as fully weight bearing even if a patient limps (Lynam 2006).

The look–feel–move examination was undertaken as follows:

Look – Both left and right legs were exposed for examination to identify obvious gross deformity, swelling, bruising, haematoma, wounds and colour. Harry had no gross deformity, swelling or wound. Bruising was present from distal to midshaft tibia; old bruising was evident along this area of both limbs. This is common in ambulant children and not a cause for concern if consistent with an active mobile child's daily activity (Merstaine *et al.* 1991)

Feel – Examination should commence in an area that is least likely to cause discomfort and pain, which can make children anxious (Oliver 1996). Harry was very anxious, and even before he was examined, he started to get upset. Every child should have a careful physical examination but only if they are relaxed and comfortable, as Harry was very upset and play was used to help to distract Harry. Harry's grandmother was asked to blow bubbles while the ENP examined his leg. Starting at the head of the fibula and working downwards, his leg was palpated, and his knee and ankle were also examined. Harry's grandparents had witnessed the fall and could concur that there were no other injuries. He was moving all other limbs easily and had no evidence of a head injury; he complained of pain only in his right leg.

While also assessing for bony tenderness, the ENP was examining for normal sensation, capillary refill and temperature of the limb to exclude neurovascular deficit. At this point, pulses of the tibial artery and dorsalis pedis were also checked (Lynam 2006).

Move – Harry had a full range of movement of both his knee and ankle, although pain was experienced on some movements of the ankle. Harry said that the pain was only in the leg and not in the ankle itself. Localising pain in children of this age group is not always accurate (Buckley 2003). Although Harry was not in much pain if left alone, the ENP offered him some analgesia, as he had none before his arrival in the ED.

Following the examination and the earlier history, the ENP decided that an X-ray of his tibia and fibula was necessary. The ENP then documented the earlier history and examination; concise documentation can provide ENPs with their own defence against allegations of misconduct and negligence (Hinchcliffe 2003). This assessment could also be supported by the use of a clinical decision support pathway (Figure 10.1) or similar evidence-based algorithm, where clinical leads in individual departments support ENPs in following a recognised pathway for particular symptoms or conditions.

On reviewing the X-ray, the ENP identified an undisplaced spiral fracture in the distal third of Harry's right tibia, more commonly described as a toddler fracture. Kinnard and Beach (2003) describes such injuries as occult non-displaced fracture of the tibia as a result of new stresses associated with ambulation applied to bone that has not previously encountered such stresses in the non-ambulant child. Although spiral fractures are often associated with non-accidental injuries (Davis 1995, Merton *et al.* 1994), other authors state that spiral fracture of the mid and lower tibia has no such implications and that isolated tibial fractures are the result of rapid linear growth and bony injury with minimal trauma (Alexander *et al.* 1987, Bays 1994). The ENP was confident that Harry's injury was accidental; bearing in mind the possibility for this being non-accidental, she discussed her findings with her clinical supervisor to explore any possible child protection issues and degree of accountability in this situation. Senior medical advice should always be sought if there is any area of concern.

This is an important issue with regard to developing advanced roles in assessment, whereas responsibility for recognition and diagnosis for key conditions are within the remit of the ENP; in recognition of the limits of her expertise and the need to ensure safe practice, she was correct in seeking the advice of the senior medical doctor.

Following discussion with the senior doctor, key factors were taken into account, such as Harry's description of events and grandparents' explanation were consistent and plausible and grandparents presented Harry early to the ED and observed interactions with the child. It was felt that there were no concerns regarding non-accidental injury (see Chapter 12 for fuller discussion of issues about child protection).

It was decided that Harry's injury could be managed conservatively as there was no displacement of the bone and Harry's pain was well controlled with simple analgesia. A long-leg plaster of Paris was applied. Harry's grandparents were given advice regarding pain control, plaster care and signs of possible complications. An outpatient fracture clinic was arranged before Harry was discharged home.

Amy Martin-Long ENP

Prescribing issues: legal, ethical and professional

Non-medical prescribing offers patients' access to health care by clinicians who are not doctors. This expansion of skill has not always been well supported. The medical profession has brought along many critics who have questioned its

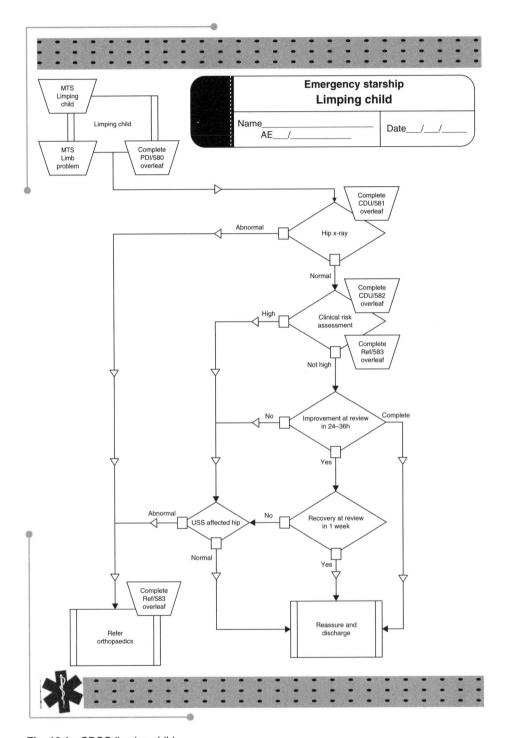

Fig. 10.1   CDSG limping child.

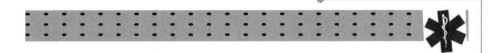

PDI/580: SUITABILITY FOR PROTOCOL DRIVEN INVESTIGATION (ALL YES)

No direct trauma to leg	Yes
Limping is the primary problem	Yes

Set 1   T, P, R, CRP, Weight, X-ray affected hip

CDU/581: X-RAY ASSESSMENT   (ANY YES)

Fracture	Yes
Avulsion	Yes
Slipped epiphysis	Yes
Perthes'	Yes

CDU/582: CLINICAL RISK ASSESSMENT for septic hip

CRP > 20	Yes
T > 38 C	Yes
Severe hip pain on examination	Yes
Tenderness over the hip	Yes

High if 2 or more positive, Low if 0 or 1 positive

Ref/583: Review clinic appointment approved	

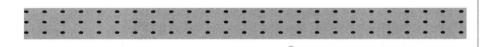

Fig. 10.1   (Continued)

safety (Horton 2002). The skill of prescribing has however been recently outlined as one of the 10 key roles by the chief nursing officer (DH 2002). NPs are individually and professionally accountable to the NMC for their prescribing (NMC 2004). Nurse prescribing must be undertaken in adherence with the NMC's Code of Professional Conduct: Standards for Conduct, Performance and Ethics in conjunction with local policies (NMC 2004). The individual nurse carries responsibility and, as such, is accountable for his/her actions. The further a professional advances in their career the more responsibility they take, both in individual interactions with people seeking health care interventions and with delegating to others. The developing skills and knowledge to become a non-medical prescriber transform the nurse into becoming a truly autonomous practitioner.

The standards make it clear that only nurses with relevant knowledge, competence, skill(s) and experience in nursing children should prescribe for children (NMC 2004). The nurse is required to act within their competency at all times and to perform reasonably as practitioners trained to the same standard within the same/similar profession with a recognised standard of competency. In terms of prescribing, this standard has been set by the medical profession, and an NP should expect her competency in prescribing to be compared with that of a doctor prescribing the same drug (Dimond 1995).

Prescribing medicines for children is challenging as it is not only the child that is being cared for but also their parent(s)/carer(s) and family. All children and young people receiving medicines should receive medicines that are safe and effective, in appropriate formulations, appropriate to their age and have minimum impact on their education and lifestyle. They should be prescribed, dispensed and administered by professionals who are well trained, informed and competent to work with children to improve health, minimise harm and any side effects associated with the drug(s). As children grow, they should be encouraged to participate and to take responsibility in the decisions about their medicines. Above all, non-medical prescribing in children should be a safe and productive prescribing experience based on the best available clinical evidence of cost-effectiveness and safety to achieve the best possible health outcomes and minimise harm and side effects.

Conclusion

The nurse consultation is an extremely satisfying learning curve, both personally and professionally. Many hurdles that lend themselves to the role of the children's advanced nurse practitioner and to nurse prescribing for children were confronted throughout the consultation process and involved the application of a whole wealth of knowledge and experience.

Maintenance of accurate records is a professional obligation, which is placed upon health professionals by their professional organisations and employer, essentially to ensure that the best and safest possible care is given to the general public. It should provide a clear record of when the patient was treated, by whom, for what reason, what management was decided and if any medication was prescribed. There should be clarity about any review dates, any further referral was made and any follow-up/instructions were given (DH 2004).

This chapter has given a comprehensive overview of the advanced nursing practitioner's role in acute settings and also given some examples of its application in practice. The following chapter expands on this and gives a picture of the broad range of such advanced and specialist roles in practice.

References

Alexander J, Fitzrandolph R and McConnell J (1987). The limping child. *Diagnostic Radiology*, 16, 229–270.

Amitage G (1999). Nursing assessment and diagnosis of respiratory distress in infants by children's nurses. *Journal of Clinical Nursing*, 8(1), 22–30.

APLS (2005). Advanced Paediatric Life Support: The Practical Approach, 4th ed. BMJ Books/Blackwells, www.blackwells.co.uk, Advanced Life Support Group.

Asthma UK (2003). *Asthma Charter*. www.asthma.org.uk.

Asthma UK (2007a). *What is Asthma?* www.asthma.org.uk.

Asthma UK (2007b). For parents: Your child has asthma. www.asthma.org.uk.

Audit Commission (1993). *Children First – A Study of Hospital Services*. London: HMSO Publications.

Baird A (2000). Crown II: The implications of nurse prescribing for practice nurses. *British Journal of Nurse Prescribing for Practice Nursing*, 5(9), 454–461.

Baird A (2001). Diagnosis and prescribing. *Primary Healthcare*, 11(5), 24–26.

Bates B (2004). *Guide to Physical Examination and History Taking*, 8th edn. Philadelphia, PA: Lippincott Williams and Wilkins.

Bays J (1994). *Conditions Mistaken for Child Abuse – Medical Diagnosis and Management*. Pennsylvania: Lea and Febiger.

Bear E (1995). Advanced practice nurses: How did we get here anyway? *Advanced Practice Nurse*, 1(1), 10–14.

Beckworth S and Franklin P (2007). *Oxford Handbook of Nurse Prescribing*. Oxford: Oxford University Press.

Benner P (1984). *From Novice to Expert – Excellence and Power in Clinical Nursing Practice*, p. 212. California: Addison Wesley.

British Medical Association (2006). *British National Formulary for Children*. England: British Medical Association Royal Pharmaceutical Society of Great Britain.

British Thoracic Society (BTS)/Scottish Intercollegiate Guidelines Network (SIGN) (2004). *British Guidelines on the Management of Asthma*. London: British Thoracic Society.

Buckley B (2003). *Children's Communication Skills from Birth to 5 Years*. London: Routledge.

Castledine G (1991). The advanced practitioner – Part 1. *Nursing Standard*, 5(44), 33–35.

Castledine G (1995). Will the nurse practitioner be a mini doctor or a maxi nurse? *British Journal of Nursing*, 4(16), 938–939.

Cox C (2004). *Physical Assessment for Nurses*. London: Blackwell Science.

CREST (2001). *Ambulatory paediatrics. Guidelines for referral and transfer. Clinical Resource Efficiency Support Team*. www.n-i.nhs.uk/crest.

Davis H and Zitteli B (1995). Childhood injuries – accidental or inflicted. *Contemporary Pediatrics*, 12(1), 94–95.

Department for Education and Skills (DfEs) and Department of Health (DH) (2004). *National Service Framework for Children, Young People and Maternity Services: Children and Young People Who Are Ill*. London: DH.

Department of Health (DH) (1976). *Fit for the Future: Report of the Court Committee on Child Health Services* (Cmnd.6884). London: HMSO.

Department of Health (DH) (1989). *Children Act*. London: HMSO, The Stationery Office.

Department of Health (DH) (1991). *Welfare of Children and Young People in Hospital*. London: HMSO.

Department of Health (DH) (1993). *Hospital Doctors; Training for the Future. Report on the Working Group or Specialist Medical Training (The Calman Report)*. London, DH.

Department of Health (DH) (1999). *Review of Prescribing Supply and Administration of Medicines* (Crown Copyright). London: DH.

Department of Health (DH) (2000a). *The National Health Service Plan. A Plan for Investment, a Plan for Reform*. London: The Stationery Office.

Department of Health (DH) (2000b). *A Health Service of All the Talents: Developing the NHS Work Force*. London: DH.

Department of Health (DH) (2001a). *Patients to Get Quicker Access to Medicines* (Press Release). London: DH.

Department of Health (DH) (2001b). *The Report of the Public Inquiry into Children's Heart Surgery at the Bristol Royal Infirmary 1984–95. Learning from Bristol*. The Stationery Office, July.

Department of Health (DH) (2002a). *Supplementary Prescribing*. London: DH.

Department of Health (DH) (2003a). *Spotting the Sick Child*, DVD, DH, OCBmedia.

Department of Health (DH) (2003b). *Getting the Right Start: National Service Framework for Children. Standard for Hospital Services*. London: DH.

Department of Health (DH) (2003c). *Report of the Neonatal Intensive Care Group*. London: HMSO Publications.

Department of Health (DH) (2004). *Extending Independent Nurse Prescribing within the NHS in England – a Guide for Implementation*, 2nd edn. London: DH.

Department of Health (DH) (2007). *Making it Better: For Children and Young People*. London: HMSO Publications.

Dimond B (1995). *Legal Aspects of Nursing*, 2nd edn. London: Prentice Hall.

Fraser LJ (1985). *Gillick v West Norfolk and Wisbech Area Health Authority and another*, 3 All ER 402 at 413.

Gray-Seiler J (2003). *Essentials of Hand Surgery, American Society for Surgery of the Hand*. Philadelphia, USA: Lippincott.

Guly H (1996). *Examination and History Taking in Emergency Medicine*. Oxford: Oxford University Press.

Hamric AB (1989). History and overview of the CNS role. In: Hamric AB and Spross JA (eds), *The Clinical Nurse Specialist in Theory and Practice*, 2nd edn, pp. 3–18. Philadelphia: W. B. Saunders.

Hamric AB and Taylor JW (1998). Role development of the CNS. In: Hamric AB and Spross JA (eds), *The Clinical Nurse Specialist in Theory and Practice*, 2nd edn, pp. 41–82. Philadelphia: W. B. Saunders.

Health Care Commission (2007). *Improving Services for Children in Hospital*. London: Commission for healthcare Audit and Inspection.

Hooker JC (1991). Change and nursing in the United Kingdom. *Journal of Advanced Nursing*, 16, pp. 253–254.

Horrocks S, Anderson E and Salisbury C (2002). Systematic review of whether nurse practitioners working in primary healthcare can provide equivalent to Drs. *British Medical Journal*, 324, 819–823.

Horton R (2002). Nurse-prescribing in the UK: Right but also wrong. *Lancet*, 359, 1875–1876.

Howard R (1997). Grasping the opportunities within evolving nursing boundaries. *Journal of Child Health*, 1(2), 81–83.

HPSS Management Plan (1999/2000 to 2001/2002).

Kinnard T and Beach R (2003). Fractured Tibia can mimic Irritable Hip. *Archives od Disease in Childhood*, 88(2), 167.

Launer J (2002). *Narrative Based Primary Care. A Practical Guide*. Oxon: Radcliffe Medical Press Limited.

Luker K, Hogg C and Austin L (1998). Decision making: The context of nurse prescribing. *Journal of Advanced Nursing*, 27, 657–665.

Lynam L (2006). Assessment of acute foot and ankle sprains. *Emergency Nurse*, 14(4), 24–33.

Maguire P and Pitceathly C (2002). Key communication skills and how to acquire them. *British Medical Journal*, 325, 697–700.

Merestein D, Cooperman D and Thompson G (1994). *Handbook of Pediatrics Limited Edition*. London: Prentice hall International (UK) London.

Merton D, Cooperman D and Thompson G (1994). *Skeletal Manifestations of Child Abuse*. Malvern, PA.

National Institute for Clinical Excellence (2002). *Principles of Best Practice in Clinical Audit*. Abing don, Oxford: National Institute for Clinical Excellence, Radcliffe Medical Press.

National Respiratory Training Centre (2006). Respiratory therapeutics. A multimedia practical learning tool for healthcare professionals. www.educationforhealth.org.uk.

NHS Management Executive (1991). *Junior Doctors: The New Deal*. London: HMSO, The Stationery Office.

Nursing and Midwifery Council (NMC) (2004). *Code of Professional Conduct: Standards for Conduct, Performance and Ethics*. London: NMC.

Nursing and Midwifery Council (NMC) (2005). *Implementation of a framework for the standard for post-registration nursing*. Council Paper ANP091105, 9 November. London, NMC.

Nursing and Midwifery Council (NMC) (2008). *Consent Nursing and Midwifery Council*. London: NMC.

Oliver RE (1996). *Guide to Examination*. Department of Child health, Dundee University.

Partridge J (2001). Children in accident and emergency: Seen but not heard? *Journal of Child Health care*, 5(2), 49–53.

Peplau H (1965). Specialisation in professional nursing. *Nursing Science*, 3, 268–287.

Report of the Platt Committee (1959). *The Welfare of Children in Hospital*. London: HMSO.

Rosenberg W and Donaldson A (1995). Evidence based medicine: An approach to problem solving. *British Medical Journal*, 310, 1122–1126.

Royal College of Nursing (RCN) (2003a). *Defining Nursing. Nursing is...* London: Royal College of Nursing.

Royal College of Nursing (2003b). *Prepaing Nurses to Care for Children and Young People*. London: RCN.

Royal College of Paediatrics and Child Health (RCPCH) (2003). *Working Time (Amendment) Regulations*. UK0212102N.

Royal College of Paediatrics and Child health (RCPCH) (2007). Services for Children in Emergency Departments. *Report of the intercollegiate Committee for Services for Children in Emergency Departments*.

Scottish Intercollegiate Guidelines Network (SIGN) (2003). Press Release: *New guidelines launched to prevent asthma deaths and cut asthma attacks and illness*.

Silverman J, Kurtz S and Draper J (1998). *Skills for Communicating with Patients*. Oxon: Radcliffe Medical Press.

Tate (2003) *The Doctors Communication Handbook*, 4th edn. Oxon: Radcliffe Medical Press.

Tortora GJ and Grabowski SR (2000). *Principles of Anatomy and Physiology*, 9th edn. USA: John Wiley and Sons.

The Victoria Climbie Inquiry (2003). The Stationery Office, January.

UKCC (1997). *Providing Nursing Care for Patients Outside Branch Specialism*, Position Statement, UKCC, March.

Wardrope J and English B (1998). *Musculoskeletal Problems in Emergency Medicine*. Oxford: Oxford University Press.

While A (2002). Practical skills: Prescribing consultation practice. *British Journal of Community Nursing*, 7(9), 469–473.

Chapter 11

Advancing Nursing Roles and Interdisciplinary Working: More Examples from Practice

Jane Hughes

Introduction

This chapter aims to further explore the scope of nurses working in advanced roles with children and their families. It hopes to demonstrate the range and potential of such advanced roles, with the use of a number of examples from practice. It should also demonstrate the degree to which many nurses in these roles work in both interdisciplinary and multidisciplinary ways.

The chapter will be broadly divided into the key areas of working for a range of specialist roles, that is, primary or community settings, secondary care, tertiary care and supra regional. Although the chapter is organised in this fashion, it aims to demonstrate how nurses in such advanced roles clearly work across these defined boundaries.

The scope and numbers of specialist nurses working with children in recent years has increased significantly, whereas 10 years ago, the number of specialist/nurses working with children was relatively small. A review of hospital websites and professional forums such as the RCN (Royal College of Nursing) and PANG (Paediatric Advanced Nurses Group) demonstrated that the development of specialist roles in various settings is gathering momentum, while not necessarily in line with the general field, these roles are clearly established in many centres.

This chapter includes a number of exemplars from the range of settings to give a flavour of some of the specialist roles and the work that they are involved in. Each exemplar will include some background to the development of the role, what professional and educational preparation that was required and the nature of the work and skills required to undertake it. In particular, the individuals will include examples of interdisciplinary and multidisciplinary and cross-boundary working. The individuals included were selected to represent a range of specialities across a number of regions; however, it is not possible to include an example of every specialism, specialist nurse or represent every part of the country, which goes some way to support the wide-ranging and developing status of advanced nursing roles with children.

Drivers for the development of specialist roles

Drivers for the development of nurses' roles have stemmed from the 1980s where the development of 'Extended and Expanded' roles were strongly debated (Wright 1989). This reflected particularly to what constituted the ethos of nursing and concerns around nurses becoming 'Mini Doctors' or technicians. However, over the past 20 years, many of the particular skills that were under question, such as the use of IV drugs and venepuncture have become an integral part of many nurses' roles, particularly with those in the general adult fields.

The *Welfare of Children in Hospital* (DH 1991) and the following audit commission 'Children First' (Audit Commission 1993) supported the need for children to be cared for by nurses trained in children's nursing; although these drivers are mainly related to general children's wards, they did help to highlight areas where children were receiving care from children's nurses who were qualified to handle children.

Significant events such as in the case of the Bristol Inquiry where children received sub-optimal care resulted in recommendations from the RCN (2001). In 'Learning the lessons', the RCN made a number of recommendations including the need for children and their families to receive appropriate child-focused services and the need to develop expert practice in specialist areas.

The Chief Nursing Officer's report in 2002 was another driver towards further development of advanced roles; Sarah Mullaley outlined 10 key roles that would be appropriate in reflecting the skills and knowledge of current qualified nurses – these included a range of skills such as ordering diagnostic investigations, admitting and discharging patients, running clinics and managing patient caseloads. These developments reflect the National Health Service (NHS) plan's (DH 2000) principle for making maximum use of the talents of the workforce and take forward recommendations from *Making a Difference* (1999b). Ultimately, the focus of such developments as illustrated in the NHS plan is to improve the patient experience. The Chief Nursing Officer (CNO) report demonstrated that nurses in such roles improve the patient experience in four key areas: speeding up access, improving treatment and care, responding to patients needs and making best use of nurses' and midwives' skills. Examples of the roles given were mainly in secondary care settings, and only 2 of the 17 illustrated roles of nurses specifically working with children and young people, namely an advanced neonatal practitioner and a parent advisor. Even in the more recent report by the RCN and Ball (2005) on 'Maxi Nurses', only 8% of such nurses surveyed were working in paediatric settings.

National Service Framework for Children and Young People

Perhaps, the greatest driver in recent years in development of specialist roles with children and young people has been in response to the National Service Framework for Children (NSF) (DH 2004b). The significant document and associated working parties stress the need to provide a better service for children and families. This support for recognition of children's unique needs has resulted in many changes such as the reorganisation of children's services, trusts, the appointment of a minister for children and increased government funding, the creation of local children and young people's networks and the development of some new local services in response to local need.

The raised awareness through the work of the national and regional children's workforces has increased the focus on the specific needs of children and helped stakeholders to plan their services to reflect the needs of children.

National Service Framework for Children, Young People and Maternity Services

Promoting health and well-being
Supporting parents and carers
Child-, young person-centred services
Growing up
Safeguarding and promoting the welfare of children
Children and young people who are ill
Children and young people in hospital
Disabled children and young people and those with complex health needs
Mental health and psychological well-being with children
Medicines
Maternity services

The NSF website is now able to demonstrate some of the outcomes of its work on the website, in particular, work with disabled children, palliative care and Child and Adolescent Mental Health Services (CAMHS) (www.dh.gov.uk/childrensnsf).

Catherine Powell (2005) outlined some of the key implications and priorities for the implementation of the NSF, and these included particular emphasis on children with disabilities and long-term conditions including those with complex needs. Another particular focus is the need for support for the increasing number of children with mental health problems.

Reorganisation of children's services

In the last 10 years the reorganisation of children's services has resulted in the past 10 years of the long-awaited development of community children's nursing (CNN)

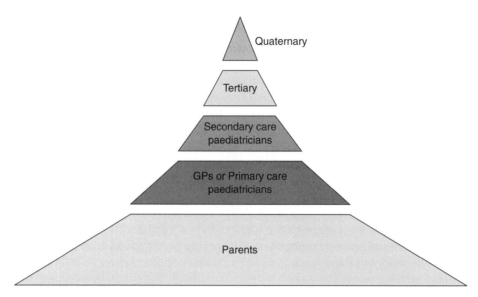

Fig. 11.1 The triangle level of service.

teams and a greater awareness that children are in need of nursing and health care support in a range of settings and not necessarily in the hospital setting. David Hall (2005a) gave a clear outline of the issues affecting children in the 21st century. He used the triangle level of service to represent this (Fig. 11.1). At the base of the triangle are the larger numbers of children who may become unwell at home for fairly short periods and do not necessarily seek any other help than from their family or local pharmacy. At the next tier, a smaller number of children require support in a community setting, often from their general practitioner (GP) or other primary sources. The next tier reflects a smaller number of children who actually require input from a secondary care setting such as the district general hospital (DGH) although not necessarily a admission; currently, the majority of children admitted to hospital stay only two nights and many staying for only one night – NSF hospital standard. The next tier reflects an even smaller number of children who require input from a tertiary setting such as a children's hospital, or regional neonatal unit where children may be more ill, stay for longer periods of time and have more complex needs. The top tier in the triangle reflects very small number of children who require care in a supra regional/fourth level or quaternary centre such as a specialist liver, renal cardiac unit.

David Hall (2005a, b) suggests that this representation of 'where children are' in the health care setting reflects the needs on the workforce of those working with children; similarly, Blair (2000) presents the issue at GPs needing to reflect community needs utilising an earlier version of the above triangle. Thus, there is a need for nurses to be involved in primary level responses to minor illness, see example by Walmsley (2006), but also being able to at the primary level offering a service for children with complex needs and mental health issues although as the above triangle, there is also a need to provide highly specialist services in tertiary centres. The recent Strengths Weakness Opportunities Threats (SWOT) analysis undertaken on behalf of the Association of Chief Children's Nurses (ACCN) suggests that there are opportunities for children and young people's nurses to cross professional boundaries and develop more flexible role that can support families in primary care settings and develop the public health role (Glasper 2005a, b).

National and local service reorganisations have also led to a need for local work forces to reflect changes such as a reduction of inpatient hospital beds and an increase in ambulatory care environments such as the review of services in the North West region, published in December 2006 (www.bestforhealth.nhs.uk). Local and regional reorganisations have often reduced access to local secondary level children services; however, primary services appropriate to children's needs are still required at a local level, hence the need for advanced nurse practitioners who can assess and manage children competently and make decisions about discharge without the need for admission to the secondary service – see Chapter 10 for more examples.

Every Child Matters

The response to the *Every Child Matters* report in 2004 is incorporated into much of the work of the NSF; however, a key driver of this report, which stemmed from the Laming report (2003) following the case of Victoria Climbie, was the need for those working with children to work more closely together and break down boundaries between disciplines, share information and support family-centred care.

The Chief Nursing Officer (2004a) stressed the need to respond to findings relating to 'fragmentation of care' and place it high on the nursing agenda. While *et al.* (2006) stresses the need to support this, particularly with regard to the growing numbers of children born with complex health needs. Such families can suffer from poor collaboration between different professionals and organisations. In the study by While *et al.* (2006), examples of cross-boundary working was identified with a number of key groups of nurses working with children with asthma, children with cancer, preschool and school children, sick neonates, children with complex needs, children in needs and troubled school age children, although she found very few examples of transdisciplinary working (nurses, midwives and health visitors working in integrated services involving different agencies).

Other recommendations of *Every Child Matters* included the need for all nurses working with children to have key skills and knowledge in child development, communicating with children and their families and training in safeguarding children (see Chapter 9, safeguarding children).

Further work of sharing information and the assessment of children in need has resulted in the Common Assessment Framework documents (http://www.everychildmatters.gov.uk/deliveringservices/caf/ Accessed 9.11.06) and Skills for Health (www.skillsforhealth.org.uk, 2006), which are being integrated into the practice of those working with children and young people. Currently, there are 13 key competencies within the children's services section of the Skills for Health framework; there are also 130 linked competencies from other frameworks (see Chapter 3).

The key competencies for those working with children and young people include the following:

- Communicate with children and young people and with those involved in their care.
- Work with children and young people to assess their health and well-being.
- Co-ordinate assessments of the health and well-being of children and young people.
- Plan, implement, monitor and review individualised care plans to meet the needs of children and young people.
- Co-ordinate and review the delivery of care plans to meet the needs of children and young people.
- Plan and implement transfer of care and discharge with children and young people and with those involved in their care.
- Plane, implement and monitor and review interventions with children and young people, and those involved in their care.
- Enable children and young people, and those involved in their care, to mange their medicines.
- Create an environment to safeguard children from abuse.
- Safeguard children and young people from abuse.
- Enable children and young people to understand their health and well-being.
- Enable children and young people to cope with changes to their health and well-being.
- Improve the services provided by practitioners to address the health and well-being needs of children and young people.

Re www.skillsforhealth.org.uk

Other influences

Clearly, these wide-ranging competencies require skills across different disciplines, and most build the basis of many nursing roles at the registered and advanced levels. Additionally, the recent integration of Agenda for Change and underpinning Knowledge and Skills Framework (KSF) (DH 2004c) used in mapping current jobs to the new pay scales brings another facet to the matching of roles at senior and advanced levels, although it has been argued that the nature of many advanced roles do not fit easily with the KSF. However, the KSF can demonstrate some of the advanced skills required for many advanced practitioners.

The RCN specialist areas (www.rcn.org.uk) and related forums support this notion of advanced levels of knowledge and competencies for specialist roles.

Chapters 10, 12 and 13 explore in some detail the skills and competencies required for these roles. The RCN produced a position statement in 2003 on the preparation of children's nurses and at the time expected to see an increase in such roles and that specific master's level programmes would have to be developed to support the development of specialist roles in children's nursing. The PaPANG clearly identifies and supports the need for specific educational programmes for those working in specialist and advanced roles with children and young people; courses are currently being developed across the country such as the Advanced Paediatric Practitioner (APNP) in Ambulatory care, MSc, at the Liverpool John Moores University. Additionally, the RCN outlines some key competencies that it has advised on with regard to the development of specialist skills with children, including chemotherapy, IV therapy, peripheral cannulation and venepuncture. Gibson *et al.* (2003) attempted to classify what could be viewed as general and specialist competencies in children's nursing, in particular, cancer care. In this extensive exercise, it was recognised that in each field or specialism, there is a hierarchy of competencies that relate to generalist and specialist nurses and that the roles could be clearly defined by using such a framework.

For the development of advanced roles in the public health, mental health and learning disability, specialisms are not discussed extensively in this chapter; however, they are addressed in Chapters 7, 8 and 9.

The evolvement of specialist roles is particularly important in supporting children and young People with the management of chronic diseases such as asthma, diabetes, epilepsy, blood and rheumatoid disorders. As mentioned previously, the needs of children with complex needs and complex conditions are also identified and demonstrated in the following sections. However, there remain areas and specialisms that are underrepresented, due to difficulties with funding and supporting children and young people with less common problems. In these cases, such children either receive care from an adult specialist nurse or are required to access services at some distance from their primary care provider.

In each of the following sections, there are accompanying case studies that aim to give an illustration of some advanced practitioners working in these areas. These will include qualifications and preparation for the role, career progression, the work involved in that specialist role, examples of interdisciplinary working and how the role might evolve in the future.

Primary care settings

As mentioned previously, the development of children's community teams has gained momentum only in recent years despite the need being identified from *Welfare of Children in Hospital* (DH 1991) and 'Health services for Children and Young people in the Community: Home and School' (House of Commons 1997). In a presentation for the community nurses forum, Karen Sinclair demonstrated some of the changes that have taken place in the provision of children's community teams – before Diana funding in 1999 in the Scottish board areas, only

4 of 15 areas had funded CCN teams, compared to the current situation of 13 of 15 areas are represented. In areas with low populations and rural areas such as Scotland and Northern Ireland (Johnston 2006, Sinclair 2006), other issues relating to the distinct problems that exist due to travel problems and isolation (see Chapter 6).

Specialist community roles specifically for children have traditionally been hard to establish due to the number of children requiring a service in a particular area; hence, many roles have been possible only from a tertiary or secondary centre as opposed to the number of specialist roles for the adult population. Similarly, until recently, respiratory and asthma care for children in the community has been taken on by adult practice nurses; in secondary care settings, however, this is a developing area, as outlined in the case study below. The development of the role of the children's respiratory nurse was in response to some local projects that are outlined in the following example, which suggested that hospital admissions and GP visits could be reduced by the input of a community children's asthma nurse.

Children's Asthma Nurse Specialist: Jane Farrell

Relevant qualifications

RGN/RSCN
A50 Diploma – Paediatric Community Nursing
Intermediate smoking cessation advisor
RETC Spirometry diploma module
NARTC – Paediatric respiratory
ENB N83 – Asthma management in acute & primary care settings

Background

Staff nurse/Sister – General medical ward specialising in cystic fibrosis, eczema and
    respiratory medicine
Paediatric asthma nurse specialist at a children's hospital
Paediatric asthma nurse specialist in the community – working on a project aimed at
    improving the quality of life and reducing morbidity of children aged 0–16 years
    with asthma, living in a defined area of Rochdale Borough. The project worked
    alongside in another demographically different area of Rochdale. The successful
    outcomes of these projects lead to the mainstream funding of two posts of paedi-
    atric asthma nursing specialist in Rochdale.

Action against asthma projects

Both projects aimed to improve the quality of life and reduce morbidity of children, 0–16 years, with asthma living in defined areas of Rochdale. It was achieved
by employing paediatric asthma nurse specialists to provide an integrated, quality asthma education service in the client's homes. The service promoted a holistic
approach to asthma management through partnership with RMBC housing, environmental health and the LEA as well as other health professionals involved in ensuring

---

the health and well-being of children with asthma. Both projects measured signifi-cant reductions in emergency care attendances at both primary and secondary care settings, morbidity of symptoms and number of days not attended school Children and parents reported satisfaction with the service they had received and improve-ments in their quality of life.

   The projects clearly identified the benefits of providing a model of care that pro-motes health education within the community setting, encourages partnership work-ing and empowers clients to seek support.

Community paediatric asthma nurse specialist role: HMRPCT

The role continues to develop following completion of the project. The service has been expanded and is now provided to whole of the Borough. Referrals are accepted from all health professionals and health partners within Rochdale Borough. The overall aim of the service is to empower the child and family to undertake self-management, at home and in school, appropriately and effectively, reducing their dependency on services and to encourage partnership working with other agen-cies. Children are taken care by the specialist nurse in their homes, and an asthma education and support programme are delivered to the family. The specialist nurses liaise between primary and secondary care to ensure a co-ordinated care pathway. Training and education is provided to health professionals and carers. A school pol-icy has been devised in conjunction with the LEA and distributed to all schools in the Borough. Asthma awareness sessions are provided to pupils and staff in schools. The specialist nurses are involved in local health promotion events. Developments for the service include the nurses undertaking the extended and supplemen-tary prescribing course to enhance the service currently offered to our clients and commissioners.

Heywood, Middleton & Rochdale PCT

The development of Diana Children's Nursing Services has evolved over the past 10 years due to funding from the Princess Diana Memorial fund. A range of services were set up to reflect a range of services. Many of these support children who have complex needs or who require palliative care. Robson and Beattie (2004) describes the aims of one particular service in Leicester to sup-port children and families with flexible negotiated care, to reduce duplication and gaps in service provision and increase the level of information and family participation. An evaluation of the service indicated that it had improved the quality of life for children and their families.

   A key aspect of the role of the children's community nurse is the ability to support children and their families in the home. The CNO report in 2004 gives further guidance as to how this role can be better integrated into wider chil-dren's services to follow the principle of following the child.

   The support of children with specific learning disabilities is addressed fur-ther in Chapter 9. However, as discussed previously, children with disabili-ties and complex needs are a specific focus of many service developments and reorganisation services, as the needs of such children have been outlined in both the NSF and the Audit Commission report in 2003.

Palliative care within primary care settings is a developing area; this is often supported by services based in local tertiary centres and sometimes supported by local hospices, although there are examples such as the Dragon Fly Team based in Stockport that was created with the support of a New Opportunities Fund bid.

Secondary level care

Secondary level care for many children in the UK will often take the form of a referral or admission to a local DGH or community hospital. Children living in large conurbation may receive secondary level care in a specific children's hospital, which may also be a tertiary centre. However, the organisation of services across the UK can mean that at the point of admission a children's inpatient bed that children are often transferred to another centre to receive the care that they need.

Local reorganisations as mentioned previously may compound this issue. The provision of specialist nurses in secondary care settings has also been affected by some of the issues that specialist nurses in primary care settings, in that funding for a specialist role had not been possible for areas where the number of children was too small to support funding for the role. However, in recent years, the number of specialist nurses in secondary care has increased, particularly in relation to asthma, diabetes and epilepsy.

Increasing incidence of childhood diabetes has led to the development of specialist children's diabetes services across the UK. The specific contribution that such nurses can make to families is outlined in a paper by Marshall *et al.* (2002). In this critical review, Marshall *et al.* stress the benefit of the support the community can give to families in enhancing education and preventing admission. Currently, many newly diagnosed children with diabetes are hospitalised for minimal periods of time, and the diabetes nurse specialist plays a key role in promoting the child and families adaptation to having a chronic illness. Marshall supports the notion that community nurses can be an effective partnership model, promote adaptation and coping and can provide a holistic model for family as opposed to a medical model. Another key area in this many specialist to roles is the education of other professionals.

Epilepsy

Paediatric epilepsy nurse specialist (as per RCN competency framework document)

I first became interested in this speciality on seeing an advertisement on the staff notice board, advertising for a 'Link Nurse' position in epilepsy, for 1 day a week.

There was also an opportunity to apply for the Diploma in Epilepsy at Leeds University. This 1 day soon increased to 2 days, and after 18 months, a full-time position was created. There was a consideration in the trust to apply for funding for a 'Sapphire Nurse', but as the trust has to secure its own funding after the 12 months of epilepsy action's financial support, this was not felt to be viable option. I completed the diploma and was promoted to paediatric epilepsy nurse specialist (PENS) after 2 years. I have been in this role for 8 years.

The first objective of the PENS nurse is to empower children, and their families, affected by epilepsy, by providing verbal and written information, support and advice about the condition from the time of diagnosis. By enabling a good understanding of their condition, and through a holistic, collaborative and co-ordinated approach to care, the PENS helps children and young people (and their families) to reach their goals of self-management. The role includes acting as a consultant and educational resource for other professionals striving towards improved, evidence-based management of epilepsy in health, social care and educational settings.

The role of the PENS will vary according to local requirements and the knowledge and experience of the individual nurse, RCN competencies (2005).

In summary, the PENS:

Will promote good practice in the assessment, diagnosis, treatment and care of children and young people with epilepsy.

Is the first point of contact, supporter and advocate for the child and family (SIGN 2005).

Is the main point of contact for GPs and other professionals, liaising between agencies and visiting at home and school when necessary to ensure continuity of care.

Supports the ongoing care of the child or young person and their family, providing specialist information, emotional support and teaching, and refers to other professionals when indicated, for example, counselling.

Provides training, education, awareness raising and advice to other professionals in schools, primary and community teams, social services, learning disability teams and so on.

Work as a key member of the multidisciplinary team, helping in the development of responsive, evidence-based, accessible and appropriate services (including nurse-led clinics) and engaging children or young people and families in service reviews and developments.

The latest clinical guidelines for managing children and young people who have epilepsy recommend that every epilepsy team should have an epilepsy nurse specialist (SIGN, 2005).

In addition to this, the National Institute for Clinical Excellence (NICE) recommends the same: 'Epilepsy specialist nurses should be an integral part of the network of care of individuals with epilepsy' (NICE 2004, p. 19).

Bernie Lee, The Tree House Stockport NHS Trust

Examples of other specialist roles in secondary care settings include specialist mental health workers, learning disability specialist nurses; however, these will be explored further in the Chapter 7 Mental health, Chapter 8 Disability. In some secondary settings, endocrine specialist nurses have also been funded.

The role of the respiratory nurse in the secondary care environment frequently covers both asthma and cystic fibrosis and other related conditions. These roles were among the first of the specialist roles that evolved in secondary care settings, and the challenge is often to sustain and develop the roles. Many of these nurses are well supported by paediatricians and who support autonomous working, such as that seen in the respiratory nurse-led clinic and outreach work to schools and local practices.

The role of the advanced neonatal nurse practitioner (ANNP) in secondary care settings is a developing area. An example of such a role is given in the next section; nurses from secondary settings are utilising similar educational programmes and with the appropriate experience are able to utilise advanced assessment and decision-making skills in the care of neonates.

It is clear that the differentiation between primary and secondary care specialist services is less clear, and many specialist workers in primary and secondary areas are crossing the boundaries that once existed. This is an important move for families and communities and is supported within the Department for Education and Skills (DfES) and Department of Health (DH) (2004) and more specifically outlined clearly by the CNO report in response to '*Every Child Matters*' in 2004 in that there is a need for effective communication between primary secondary and tertiary settings.

Tertiary

The tertiary setting for children and young people will reflect a different experience for children and young people compared to that for the adult patient; this reflects the particular nature of specialist care available for children in the UK. The provision of tertiary care again will vary due to the particular demographic aspects of a particular location. A child living in large urban locations is likely to benefit from at least one specialist children's tertiary centre as in Manchester, Birmingham, London, Bristol, Leeds and so on, and the specialist services provided will cover a range of specialisms. However, a child in a smaller town located some distance from a specialist tertiary centre may be more reliant on secondary care in the local area, and accessing specialist services will require travelling 50 miles or more to a specialist centre. Children and their families in a rural setting such as those in parts of Wales and Scotland face a unique challenge in that specialist services may not be accessible without an overnight stay, and any specialist services offered may also require some travel and liaison with secondary and primary services.

Many tertiary settings offer a range of services covering specialities such as diabetes (see the following case study), neonatology, intensive care epilepsy, cancer, burns, pain, cystic fibrosis, intravenous services, ear nose and throat, orthopaedic, haematology, neurology, imaging and in some areas of genetic services.

Examples of nurses working in some of these areas are included below. In a number of specialisms, tertiary centres have been able to set up a team of specialist nurses for a particular area, whereas in the primary and secondary settings, specialist nurses are often working independently without the support of nurses in their specialist area.

Diabetes

Diabetic nurse specialist: Carole Gelder

As a registered sick children's nurse, I first specialised in paediatric nephrology at Great Ormond Street Hospital. An interest in improving standards and supporting staff led to the development of a paediatric nephrology course and a subsequent secondment to do a PGDE/MSc in Health Professional Education. During this time, an opportunity arose to develop specialist clinical skills as a children's diabetes nurse specialist. At this time, the role was primarily managing children with Type 1 diabetes, but over the years, the role has expanded to include some rarer forms of diabetes that require highly specialist clinical skills such as Type 2, cystic fibrosis-related diabetes (CFRD), steroid induced, maturity onset diabetes of the young (MODY) and neonatal diabetes.

In 2002, the insulin pump therapy (continuous subcutaneous insulin infusion, CSII) service in Leeds was started. However, with CSII use in the UK, considerably lower than in Europe and the US and with a limited evidence base, there were few resources to draw on. Consequently, practice and service needed to be developed, standards still needed to be set, policies and information devised. This leading edge work soon became one of my main responsibilities as clinical lead and co-ordinator for the insulin pump therapy service in Leeds. By 2006, we had an established pump service with over 60 children on insulin pumps, ranging from babies of just 2 weeks through to teenagers. Skills in CSII are not confined to one person; all in the team are proficient autonomous practitioners, and paediatric ward staff also have developed knowledge and skills so that families can access the ward for support 24 hours a day.

The most challenging but satisfying group of patients clinically have been babies on insulin pumps. Before CSII it was not possible to achieve optimal blood glucose control in this age group due to dramatic variation in blood glucose, which often causes irritability in babies or still worse hypoglycaemic fits. Insulin pumps enable very small doses of insulin to be given, which can be matched to the individual's unique physiological needs. This has brought about real change to the management of this age group, and anecdotal reports suggest a dramatic improvement in lifestyle for the families involved.

In view of the need to develop advanced clinical skills in CSII coupled with masters level academic skills (RCN guidance 2006), an insulin pump therapy module was developed in collaboration with a higher education provider to respond to this challenge. The course is multidisciplinary and equally accommodates paediatric and adult health care professionals with the aim of creating a seamless transition between services and greater understanding of one and other's roles within teams. With a philosophy of empowerment running through this module, the aim was to also facilitate the translation of this approach into clinical interventions with children and young people.

This role as clinical lead for CSII has also led to participation on the DH insulin pump working group and as a committee member of Pump Management for Professionals (PUMP). These groups have provided a wide range of opportunities such as raising awareness nationally, offering support through networks, generating

---

new solutions, developing a toolkit for commissioners of pump therapy and a core curriculum for pump therapy education for service users and professionals.

Further opportunities have also arisen to review articles for academic journals, contribute to this book, another on insulin pump therapy and take up a post as a lecturer/practitioner on the CSII module.

Leeds

Neonates

Advanced neonatal nurse practitioner: Viv Hall

I am a registered general nurse and also a midwife. It was my midwifery training that gave me my first introduction to neonates and I was hooked. After gaining my specialist neonatal qualification (ENB 405) and moving to a regional neonatal intensive care unit, I further developed my theoretical knowledge and clinical skills by undertaking the R23 module. This module, which formed part of my BSc, taught skills such as cannulation, intubation, blood gas interpretation and ventilator management.

Working in a regional centre involves caring for the smallest and sickest infants, using the newest and specialised treatments available. As these infants may be born at their local hospital, they require transport into the regional centre. My interest in neonatal transport developed and an opportunity arose for a specialist practitioner to develop a dedicated neonatal transport team (UKCC Scope of Professional Practice 1992, TINA Report 1995).

The aim of the service was to provide a multidisciplinary team who were highly trained and experienced in the problems of neonatal transport that could impact positively on neonatal outcomes. The development of the service has grown from a team that provided transport for one hospital to an independent specialist provider for the network that includes 13 hospitals.

The transport service invested in my ANNP training (MSc) and subsequently I was employed as the first ANNP and transport team leader. Although the ANNP's initial responsibility is to the team, we work concurrently on the neonatal intensive care unit alongside the SHOs and registrars. This dual role enables us to maintain our expertise and provides supervision and mentorship opportunities. Our role is predominantly clinically based although we have commitments to education, research and development, management and clinical governance issues.

The implementation of the ANNPs in neonatal units varies greatly and is currently developing according to the needs of the individual units; however, the introduction of ANNP roles allows for further growth and development for nurses who wish to remain clinically based rather than follow the management/education routes that traditionally were the only options for senior staff.

References

Scope of Professional Practice (1992) UKCC.
TINA (Transport of Neonates in Ambulances) Report (1995) MDA.

To ensure children and families receive a good quality and seamless service, it is important that tertiary centres liaise closely with referring secondary care centres and primary care services to ensure care is provided in a consistent manner and that families do not suffer from problems with communication regarding care (see NHS experience – e.g. Cass 2006). Historical hierarchical boundaries between tertiary and secondary settings are no longer acceptable in the light of the current climate; the CNO report (2004) supports this argument. Tertiary care centres must liaise appropriately with secondary and primary care givers to ensure children and young people receive seamless and high quality care. These type of working partnerships are highlighted in some of the examples below.

Funding for epilepsy and palliative care specialist nurses from charitable bodies such as Sapphire, Macmillan or CLIC Sargent has been made possible in a number of locations across the country and can be observed in a number of tertiary and secondary care centres; the support of charities in providing funding for such nurses is invaluable as the establishment and continuation of many such posts would not have been possible without the support of these charitable organisations.

Jane Hunt in 1995 outlined the role of the specialist oncology community, which has been developed to support to care for children and young people with cancer and leukaemia. Theses specialist nurses are primarily based in tertiary centres in the UK, although some are based in secondary care settings. A major source of funding for such nurses was from charities; of the 43 interviewed at the time, 9 were funded by the NHS, 10 were funded by Cancer and Leukaemia in Childhood, 5 were funded by Macmillan and 19 by other charities.

In some tertiary centres, it has been possible to establish a team of specialists. In the case of cancer, some units have children's oncology nurse specialists, bone marrow transplant specialists and outreach roles, and in some cases specialist teenager cancer nurses.

Unique to many services are 24-hour on-call services offering specialist support to children and their families, including palliative care and prescribing of key medication.

Paediatric oncology specialist

Viv Allison is an experienced nurse who currently works as Paediatric Oncology Outreach Nurse Specialist (POONs) in Newcastle. Viv qualified as an SRN in 1975 and RSCN in 1991. She worked in various settings before qualification as a children's nurse, which included being a staff nurse on a children's surgical ward, night sister in a DGH, staff nurse on several adult wards and a recovery area. Once qualified as an RSCN, she worked as a staff nurse in a general paediatric ward of a DGH before

taking up the post as a senior staff nurse on several wards in a tertiary centre cater-
ing for children and young people with neurological disorders, head injuries, general paediatric conditions, immunology disorders and neuro-oncological problems.
Her interest was in nursing children and young people with cancer, and she then
moved, as a senior staff nurse, to work in the child and teenage oncology unit. She
soon became the ward sister on the children's ward of this unit before moving into
the POONs team five years ago.

The current POONs team consists of the four whole time equivalent posts of four
full-time posts. The team offer a 24-hour on-call service to patients and their families who have complex needs or who require palliative care at home. The nurses are
a key contact for the families and they liaise and communicate with local primary
health care teams, paediatric oncologists, social workers, teachers, hospital nursing
staff, occupational therapists, physiotherapists and pharmacists to co-ordinate an
appropriate package of care. The role is a demanding one, requiring the nurses to
have excellent communication and interpersonal skills to support families in very
challenging and distressing situations. The nurses need to have the knowledge, skills
and confidence to manage the symptoms and problems that the children, young people and their families may face in the terminal stages of their disease. The care is
managed in conjunction with consultant colleagues and other members of the multidisciplinary team, but the POONs nurses are often working alone with the families
when problems or new symptoms have arisen. Further education and training in
relation to palliative care, bereavement care and nurse prescribing are all important
in the personal and professional development of the nurses working in this field.
Enabling children and young people to die in their place of choice, usually their own
home, is very important, and the POONs team and particularly the 24-hour on-call
service provides support for families to enable this to take place.

Support for bereaved children and families is a another evolving area;
many services have developed in response to local need, as in many services in regional centres where bereaved parents seek support following the
death of their child. The national picture in relation to bereavement services for parents and children remains patchy [Rolls and Payne (2003)], and
many of these services rely heavily on support from voluntary sectors such
as Macmillan, Cruse, Child Bereavement Trust, Compassionate friends and
Marie Curie.

In the community, support for bereaved children comes in many forms, from
health school nurses or specialist bereavement services, in schools, in the form of
pastoral care from education workers or school nurses. Where children develop
more significant needs following their bereavement, children may require help
from CAMHS, or children may seek help through the voluntary sector including hospices. Provision is patchy and variable across the country, and nurses
with a particular interest/skill in this area have responded to needs; however,
this remains an area that does not receive universal support and funding from
health and social care providers.

Continence

Nurse specialist stoma care and promotion of continence: Pat Coldicutt

Alder Hey Children's Hospital

Qualifications include SRN, RSCN, NNEB, Ba Hons, DPSN, ENB 998, ENB 216, Specialist practice module, ENB N110 (counselling).

I have been in post for 14 years and before this I was the nursing process coordinator that involved teaching staff and implementing the nursing process. I realised my lack of knowledge when I was appointed in this role, and therefore, I applied to complete a nursing diploma and first degree after that. These have helped me a great deal and my confidence and knowledge has grown over the past years. I am not ashamed to say that I still learn something new each day, be it a tip from a parent of a child. I do learn a lot from them and I enjoy the rapport we build.

Some of the patients that I deal with are referred shortly after birth with conditions such as imperforate anus; initially, the family requires support after the initial diagnosis as this is often is a very difficult time for parents especially when the baby they have longed for is born with an abnormality. Often, it is the father whom we deal with in the first hours after birth. I work closely with the surgical team, anaesthetists and the paediatrician. Such interdisciplinary work is important so as to ensure that the family has a clear understanding of what the condition involves and the proposed plan for treatment including possible complications.

My role is also around supporting ward staff who teach the parents the care of colostomies and other stoma care.

Another aspect of my role includes the support of families whose children suffer from bowel problems such as soiling and constipation; this can significantly affect the child's quality of life. My role may include support and advice for dealing with incontinence and also teaching about giving medicines and in some cases bowel washouts.

Continued involvement with the family over a long period of time can allow the specialist nurse an appreciation of the concerns and anxieties that families may experience. Their main role at this point is to provide support and to help them through their child's journey and frequent hospital visits. This gives a great insight into the understanding and the individual family's needs. Specific skills include the ability to encourage parents talk about their fears, hence really good listening skills. You need to be able to talk to the child in a language it understands and likewise with the parents.

I also work with play specialists who can play a key role, various aids such as dolls, bags, pictures of real patients and stomas can be utilised in preparing children and families.

Other issues involved in the support of the child and family include support for the child in school. Education staff can be supported to deal with children's stoma and continence needs although often special carers' are required.

Rheumatology

The role of the paediatric rheumatology clinical nurse specialist

Liz Hutchinson
Clinical Nurse Specialist
Nottingham Children and Young Peoples' Rheumatology Service

Background

I have been in post since 2002. My career pathway can be summarised as RGN training, RSCN training, 18 months of paediatric intensive care experience, district nurse training and 13 years as a children's community nurse, predominantly with an oncology remit. Later, I managed the entire children's community nursing service in Nottingham where I supported our consultant paediatric rheumatologist in building a business case for this post. Once funding was secured from the primary care trust and the recruitment process initiated, I decided to apply for the post. My previous experience provided me with many of the skills needed for this role; therefore, my learning has been around acquiring disease-specific knowledge. Without a paediatric rheumatology nursing qualification, I have enhanced my practice through:

- Working alongside paediatric rheumatology colleagues.
- Attending paediatric rheumatology meetings locally, nationally and internationally.
- Networking with paediatric rheumatology colleagues.
- MSc in Advanced Nursing Practice – Assignments tailored to rheumatology (e.g. immunology).

Role

Paediatric and adolescent rheumatology services are generally provided within tertiary centres by a dedicated multidisciplinary team. Working with the lead medical and therapy staff, I have led the strategic development and commissioning of the clinical networks for rheumatology and CFS/ME, in partnership with the patients, their families/carers and professionals from all relevant agencies. This involves continuous review of patient pathways within the context of advances in therapeutic care, evidence-based guidelines and NHS guidance for rheumatology [1–11]. I provided expert advice, education, training and support for patients and staff within the clinical network. I have implemented care pathways, nurse-led initiatives and improved links with primary care, secondary care, education, social services and the voluntary agencies. The transitional needs of young people have been addressed through co-working with my adult colleagues.

Using my specialist knowledge and resources, I empower medical, nursing and allied health professionals to facilitate appropriate care for the children and young people. I co-ordinate all hospital and community care for children and young people under the remit of the paediatric rheumatology service. Many of these children are under shared care arrangements, where I support the local teams to manage their care.

On a more practical level, I continue to work directly with patients acting as their advocate as they journey through their illness trajectory. Engaging patients to take treatments often with unpleasant side effects requires all my powers of persuasion and negotiation. I consider that I am pivotal to ensuring that patients are cared for in a safe and timely manner by the multi-professional team. Furthermore,

---

I am the link to the provision of care in the community liaising with schools, nurseries, social services, pharmacy home care companies and voluntary agencies. For the families, I am the main point of contact and I can be accessed by telephone or email.

Advances in the care of rarer diseases, such as in paediatric rheumatology conditions, require international collaboration. To improve disease outcomes, and quality of life of patients, I am involved in collaborating at an international and national level with paediatric rheumatology research and audit.

This post is diverse and varied; the learning is ongoing and as new treatments emerge, my role of the nurse will continues to evolve. None of the above is possible without the support and encouragement of my colleagues within the rheumatology team, particularly my clinical nurse specialist (CNS) colleague.

Cardiac

The role of the Paediatric Cardiac Liaison Sister

Catherine Harrington, Bristol Children's Hospital

The role of the Cardiac Liaison Sister is so varied across the whole of the UK. We all have such different job descriptions, roles and responsibilities. Many have changed their title to 'Specialist nurse'. I decided to keep the 'Liaison' title, as I felt it best described what my role was, even though I encompass a specialist background, skills and knowledge.

I will discuss the role of the Paediatric Cardiac Liaison Sister (PCLS) in Bristol, as it is at the moment, and plans for the future of this service.

My background is paediatric intensive care. The reason why such a post interested me was the family involvement and support. I would be the common link to the child and their family during their journey from diagnosis to surgery and treatment. Sadly, some of my work is caring for these children and families who have only palliative treatments and unfortunately, at times, provide bereavement counselling.

As part of my job specification, the PCLS should hold or working towards a degree. This was necessary due to the recent 'banding' that kept this role in line with a ward sister.

My paediatric ITU course and qualification in Counselling helped my application. I am now working towards my BSc (Hons) in Child Health and plan to continue towards my MSc in Clinical Assessment, involving prescribing. The reasons why will come apparent.

My ethos for the PCLS is to provide a specialist service to those affected with congenital or acquire heart disease, providing support, information and advice. This will start at the time of diagnosis, including anti-natal diagnosis, through to their treatment and to the transition to adulthood.

The development of the service has been huge. I work closely within a large multi-professional team, involving medical, nursing, psychology and play specialists, not just within the specialist centre but with the whole of the South West.

Nurse specialists have similar roles, such as working closely with other agencies such as schools and other specialist teams. However, two roles that I have developed in the five years of being in post are the following:

Providing support and education of home management and monitoring of warfarin. Instigating the purchase of equipment, liaising with GPs and local hospitals and management of dosage through the phone.

Pre-operative assessment, holding a weekly clinic, essentially to lessen anxiety and answer questions, but now becoming more clinically focused. This I see as a developing role for the PCLS as reduction of doctor's hours could mean the development of an advanced nurse practitioner/nurse consultant, clinically assessing the child and obtaining consent.

The Department of Health (2001) and subsequent studies have suggested that there should be at least six PCLS per specialist centre. I have been working full time by myself for 10 months.

It can be a very stressful role as you have so many responsibilities and families have so many needs, but I now have some of my anti-natal babies starting school and I am included in those and other special times, which makes all the stress and at times the heartache all worth it.

Supra regional

Supra regional or quaternary services may or may not be combined with a traditional tertiary centre, and often a centre may offer a mix of what may be considered tertiary and supra regional services. This may be based on historical development of a specialist service in a particular location; alternatively, the tertiary aspect may be fully combined within the supra regional centre.

The Hospital for Sick Children in London offers many services at a supra regional level and some at tertiary levels. As the basis for the Institute of Child Health, it aims for be a hub of knowledge for professionals and children and families (www.ich.ucl.co.uk). Its offers information and support to other centres, and the web site currently links to other tertiary children's centres across the country.

Examples of some supra regional services offered include specialist cardiac – Alder Hey, GOS, Bristol, Birmingham; liver – Birmingham; neonatal surgery – Manchester, Birmingham, London.

As seen earlier, there is a need for many of these services to provide a service that reaches out to children and families wherever they are, even though they are situated within tertiary and supra regional centres. The following example of the cleft lip and palate service demonstrates a varied role that requires a specialist to visit families at birth at various points further along to support families. It also involves providing education and support for professionals caring for such children and families both at pre-registration and in clinical practice. A unique aspect of this service is a joint clinic that provides multidisciplinary services for the child and family in one location.

Regional cleft lip and palate service: North West of England

Jacob was a 3-week-old baby who was readmitted, at a weekend, onto a paediatric ward at his local DGH following his collapse at home. Paediatric examination revealed a cleft palate, and this young baby and his family were referred to the Regional Cleft Lip & Palate On-Call Service staffed by clinical nurse/health visitor specialists (CNS).

An assessment visit was arranged within 24 hours of the referral (National Standard, CSAG) in collaboration with the paediatric and nursing staff where the diagnosis of a cleft palate was confirmed. Additional features of severe Pierre Robin sequence were identified by the CNS, a combination of micrognathia and glossoptosis causing marked upper airway obstruction.

On further examination, in supine, both tracheal tug and an intercostal recession were noted, and blood gasses, ordered by the CNS, revealed raised pCO_2 of 10.5 KPa. Although these symptoms were reduced by placing the baby in a lateral position, the CNS advised the placement of a nasopharyngeal tube to relieve the upper airway problems and a nasogastric tube for nutrition. As this particular hospital had not used this airway recently, the CNS was able to teach staff to measure, place and secure the tube comfortably in place. This procedure was observed by a number of medical and nursing staff as, in this situation, it is important that resident staff are confident in the management and replacement of the airway. A management plan was agreed in that the airway would remain in place, nutrition would be provided through a nasogastric tube in conjunction with non-nutritive sucking and oral stimulation, and blood gasses would be monitored until stable and within normal limits. Throughout the procedure and planning, Jacob's mother was present and a phased training for herself and community paediatric staff was put into place. Discharge planning with the correct equipment meant Jacob was discharged home within 10 days of admission into the care of his mother. Weekly support and forward planning was provided by the CNS in conjunction with the local primary health care team, and Jacob remained in the care of his mother. With growth, weight gain and oromotor development, these problems gradually resolved and a planned removal of the nasopharyngeal airway was arranged by the CNS as an inpatient on the paediatric ward. Jacob is now 4½ months old and shows no evidence of upper airway obstruction. He enjoys oral feeding and no longer relies on nasogastric tube feeding. His mother is proud of her achievements and feels that she has been well supported, both practically and emotionally throughout this period.

The CNS is a core member of the multidisciplinary teams working within the nine regional centres throughout England and Wales. They work autonomously providing immediate and continuing holistic care to families affected by facial clefts, and their associated anomalies, in partnership with local service services. The CNS has a health visitor and/or paediatric nurse professional qualification and is educated to degree level. Additional counselling, leadership and teaching qualifications are required, and a 6-month specialist programme is undertaken at level 3. Postgraduate education to masters/clinical doctorate is encouraged to enable the nurse to assimilate and apply a wide range of knowledge and understanding to clinical practice, teaching, audit and research.

Trish Bannister, Specialist Health Visitor

Conclusion

This chapter has demonstrated the potential range of the many new roles and recent possibilities for career progression working in specialist areas with children and young people. For nurses working with children and young people with a special interest in a speciality, it is demonstrated that there is clear potential for such nurses to become experts in their field and to work autonomously supported within their speciality by other professionals.

These roles clearly have a requirement not only for knowledge of the specialist, but also for enhanced decision-making skills and further academic study to consolidate such roles.

There are also growing support networks such as RCN and PANG across the country, thus enforcing the key roles that such nurses can play in supporting children young people and their families. The development of cross-boundary and interdisciplinary work is another positive area that has evolved over the recent years and supports recent recommendations, although as While *et al.* (2006) illustrates that children's nurses have a great potential to work in a more interdisciplinary way. There are still some regions where it is more difficult to establish specialist roles due to funding problems or logistical issues due to location and difficulties with the rural nature.

References

Audit Commission (1993). *Children First: A Study of Hospital Services.* London: Her Majesty's Stationery Office.

Audit Commission (2003). *Services for disabled children and their families.* www.auditcommision.gov.uk.

Blair M (2000). Taking a population perspective on child health. *British Medical Journal,* 83, 7–9.

Department for Education and skills (DfES) and Department of Health (DH) (2004). National Service Framework for Children, Young People and Maternity Services: Children and Young People Who Are Ill. London: DH.

Department of Education and Skills (2005). *Common Core of Skills and Knowledge for the Children's Workforce.* HMSO London.

Department of Education and Skills (2006). *Common Assessment Framework for Children and Young People.* London: DFES.

Department of Health (DH) (1991). *Welfare of Children in Hospital.* London: Her Majesty's Stationery Office.

Department of Health (DH) (1999a). *The NHS Plan.* London: DH.

Midwifery and Health Visiting Contribution to Health and Health Care. London: DH.

Department of Health (DH) (2000). Framework for the Assessment of Children in Need and Their Families. London: HMSO.

Department of Health (DH) (2001). *The Report of the Public Inquiry into Children's Heart Surgery at the Bristol Royal Infirmary 1984–95: Learning from Bristol.* London: HMSO, The Stationery Office.

Department of Health (DH) (2002). *Developing Key Roles for Nurses and Midwives: A Guide for Managers – Chief Nursing Officer*. DH Publications London.

Department of Health (DH) (2004a). *The Chief Nursing Officer's Review of the Nursing, Midwifery and Health Visiting Contribution to Vulnerable Children and Young people*. DH Publications London.

Department of Health (DH) (2004b). *National Service Framework for Children, Young People and Maternity Services: Executive Summary*. www.dh.gov.uk/childrensnsf.

Department of Health (DH) (2004c). *Knowledge and Skills Framework*. www.modern.nhs.uk/agendaforchange

Gibson F, Fletcher M and Casey A (2003). Classifying general and specialist children's nursing competencies. *Journal of Advanced Nursing*, 44(6), 591–602.

Glasper EA (2005a). On behalf of the association of Chief Children's Nurses. *The Future of Pre-registration Child and Young peoples Nursing Preparation, a Swot Analysis*, ACCN.

Glasper EA (2005b). Preparation of children and young peoples nurses in the future. *National Service Framework for Children, Young People and Maternity Services: Initiatives, Implications and Implementation*, The source Sheffield November 2005, the University of Sheffield.

Hall D (2005a). The NSF for Children: An Overview, Implications of the NSF for Children's Nursing Practice. *National Service Framework for Children, Young People and Maternity Services: Initiatives, Implications and Implementation*, The source Sheffield November 2005, The University of Sheffield.

Hall D (2005b). Primary care for children in the 21st century. *British Medical Journal*, 330, 430–431.

House of Commons (1997). *Health Services for Children and Young people in the Community: Home and School*, House of Commons.

Hunt J (1995). The paediatric oncology community nurse specialist: The influence of employment location and funders on models of practice. *Journal of Advanced Nursing*, 22(1), 126–133.

Johnston P (2006). *The challenges of providing an acute children's community nursing service in Northern Ireland – Royal College of Nursing Children's Community Nursing Conference 2006*. www.rcn.org.uk.

Marshall M, Flemming E, Gillibrand W and Carter B (2002) Adaptation and negotiation as an approach to care in paediatric diabetes specialist nursing practice: A critical review. *Journal of Clinical Nursing*, 11, 421–429.

NHS (2006). *Making it better for children, young people, parents and babies consultation*. www.bestforhealth.nhs.uk/page.asp?branchchid=CHILDADULT (accessed 9 November 2006).

Powell C (2005). Implications of the NSF for Children's Nursing Practice. *National Service Framework for Children, Young People and Maternity Services: Initiatives, Implications and Implementation*, The source Sheffield November 2005, The University of Sheffield.

Robson A and Beattie A (2004). Diana Children's Community Service and service co-ordination. *Child: Care, Health and Development*, 30(3), 233–239.

Rolls L and Payne S (2003). Childhood bereavement services: A survey of UK provision. *Palliative Medicine*, 17, 423–432.

Royal College of Nursing (RCN) (2001). *Learning the Lessons – a Summary of the RCN's Response to the Bristol Inquiry*. London: RCN.

Royal College of Nursing (RCN). *Forums and Specialist Zones*. www.rcn.org. (accessed September 2006).

Royal College of Nursing (RCN) and Ball J (2005). *Maxi Nurses. Advanced and Specialist Roles*. London: RCN.

Scottish Intercollegiate Guidelines Network (SIGN) (2005). Diagnosis and management of epilepsies in children and young people. www.sign.ac.uk

Sinclair K (2006). The Scottish Perspective of the Community Children's Nursing service. *Royal College of Nursing Children's Community Nursing Conference 2006*. www.rcn.org.uk.

The Victoria Climbié Inquiry (2003). *Report of an Inquiry by Lord Laming Presented to the Parliament by the Secretary of State for Health and the Secretary for the Home Department by Command of Her Majesty*, HMSO. www.skillsforhealth.org.uk (2006).

Walmsley C (2006). Setting up a minor illness and injury service for children up to five years. *Paediatric Nursing*, 18(3), 30–33.

While A, Murgatroyd B, Ullmand R and Forbes A (2006). Nurses', midwives' and health visitors' involvement in cross boundary working within child health services. *Child, Care, Health and Development*, 32(1), 87–99.

Wright S (1989). Expanding the nurse's role. *Nursing Standard*, 36(3), 44.

Chapter 12

Careers in Research and Education

Alison Twycross

Introduction

Nursing career pathways in research and education are often not defined. Indeed when writing this chapter, I found very little information to support what I was saying. In the light of this much of what is written in this chapter is my perspective on what is required. In this chapter, I have set out to provide information about the different career pathways that are open to children's nurses in research and education. I have provided an indication of the qualifications, experience and skills required to enter each of these pathways as well as providing guidance on the steps you need to take to move along a given career pathway. I will start by looking at career pathways in nurse education and then discuss a number of distinct research career pathways. Information about some of the support networks for those working in education and research is also provided.

Career pathways in education

Becoming a nurse educator

Most nurses move into their first teaching job following a number of years working in clinical practice. An interest in education and learning and supporting students are usually qualities demonstrated by those who wish to take the first step towards a career in nurse education. Indeed, two of the main prerequisites for a lecturer post are to be on the Nursing and Midwifery Council (NMC) register and to have the relevant clinical expertise. Some experience of teaching is also essential, whether ward based or in the school of nursing, as is having a degree. Indeed, most schools of nursing expect teaching staff to have a master's degree. Evidence of some experience of undertaking research and/or audit is essential and publications and conference presentations desirable. If you do not have a teaching qualification, you will be expected to undertake one in your first academic year working in the university. For the lecturer supporting students studying children and young people's (CYP) nursing, an awareness of the current issues around pre-registration training for branch, is also important (see Chapter 2).

The title of your first post in education will depend on which university you are employed by as different universities have slightly different job titles (Table 12.1). As a general rule, the *old* English and Welsh universities and all the Scottish universities use one set of titles, whereas the *new* English and Welsh universities use another. As most nurses move into their first job in education after a number of years in clinical practice, they usually start their teaching career at the lecturer B/senior lecturer level.

Traditionally, when working in a university academic, staff engage in research and scholarly activity for 20% of their time (1 day a week). Within nursing, teaching loads are often greater than in other disciplines, and this does not always happen. However, I have found that if you manage your diary effectively and plan ahead, it is usually possible to have a day a week to work on such activities. Definitions of scholarly activity vary. The University of Hertfordshire (2006) defines research and scholarly activity as:

- The production of books and monographs.
- Contributions to books, articles and conference papers.
- Creative and original work in all media.
- Professional updating and personal academic development.

The lecturer–practitioner role

An alternative option to a full-time teaching role is to become a lecturer–practitioner. A lecturer–practitioner spends half their week working in the university and the other half working in clinical practice. Lecturer–practitioner roles vary from place to place, and there is no standard job description. Sometimes, lecturer–practitioners are used to run post-registration courses such as paediatric intensive care courses and are seconded from their clinical appointment to do so. Alternatively, a lecturer–practitioner may be appointed jointly by the clinical area and university (although if this is the case, your contract will usually be held by one employer and you will have an honorary contract with the

Table 12.1 Alternative job titles

'Old' English and Welsh Universities and Scottish Universities	'New' English and Welsh Universities
Lecturer A	Lecturer
Lecturer B	Senior lecturer
Senior lecturer	Principal lecturer

other). To become a lecturer–practitioner, you need to have excellent clinical skills, teaching experience, leadership skills and a degree (preferably a master's degree).

If you are not sure whether a career in education is for you, a lecturer–practitioner role *keeps your options open*, allowing you to get a feel for education but keeping your foot firmly in clinical practice too. However, although the lecturer–practitioner role does support the integration of theory and practice, there are also some issues that you need to consider when deciding whether this is the role for you. Rhead and Strange (1996) found for example that lecturer–practitioners felt that they were serving two masters and that there was an expectation of giving 100% to each, whereas Leigh *et al.* (2005) found that there was often a lack of collaboration between the hospital and university, particularly at first. These findings echo my own experiences and illustrate the need for such appointments to be well thought through. One strategy I used was to set joint objectives and to have a review meeting every 3 months at which my managers from both organisations were present.

Moving along the educational career pathway

The majority of teaching staff within a school of nursing will be at the lecturer B/senior lecturer level. Sometimes, nurses move to other universities to a post at the same grade to gain experience in another area. However, there are two ways to get promoted to senior lecturer/principal lecturer. The first is to apply for a post in another institution; the second is to apply for internal promotion. When considering internal promotions and appointments at senior lecturer/ principal lecturer level, universities look at candidate's contributions in three key areas:

- Teaching.
- Research.
- Administration, development and enterprise.

To be promoted or offered a senior lectureship/principal lectureship, you would be expected to perform excellently in two of these areas and well in the other area. In relation to teaching, the individual would be expected to demonstrate substantial leadership in the full range of pedagogic activities. Kingston University for example look for evidence of:

1. Acknowledged leadership and future leadership potential, helping and guiding others in the planning, delivery and assessment of teaching and learning.
2. A significant contribution to the development of teaching and learning.
3. Proven excellence in the delivery and assessment of teaching and learning.

(Kingston University 2001)

An individual's contribution to research would be expected to include the following:

1. Proven contribution to research in a particular discipline.
2. Good record of publication of original work.
3. Success in obtaining funds for research projects.
4. Successful supervision of research projects/students.

(Kingston University 2001)

In relation to administration, development and enterprise, an individual would be expected to demonstrate:

1. Responsibility for a substantial block of work essential to a course or programme. This may include managing a particularly significant aspect or co-ordinating major elements of the activity. Such work must carry a substantial level of responsibility.
2. Substantial management responsibility, including budget management, for a block of work that is not necessarily directly related to the courses or programmes, but which may include school of faculty-wide responsibility.
3. A combination of the above. A role involving both substantial duties relating to a course or programme and substantial school or faculty-wide responsibility.
4. Entrepreneurial activities particularly outreach to business and industry.

(Kingston University 2001)

The use made of the research and scholarly activity time is key to gain the skills and expertise required for promotion.

Becoming a head of school

Once you have been a principal/senior lecturer for a number of years, you may want to consider becoming a head of school. To become a head of school, you will need to demonstrate that you:

- Have management and leadership skills.
- Have management experience.
- Have a breadth of thinking about educational processes.
- Have knowledge of the evidence underpinning educational processes.
- Are able to think strategically.
- Are able to move things forward (i.e. that you are a risk taker).

All heads of school will have a master's degree and a professional nursing qualification; many heads of school now have doctorates. Experience of managing budgets is desirable but not essential.

Becoming a dean

The next step on the career pathway and one that many nurse educators do not aspire to is the dean of a faculty. To become a dean, you will need to demonstrate that you:

- Have the analytical skills to deal with complex situations.
- Have people management skills.
- Have knowledge and understanding of learning and educational processes.
- Have knowledge and experience of strategies for improving quality.
- Experience of financial management.
- Able to work in partnership with other schools and organisations.
- Knowledge and understanding of current policy in health and higher education across the UK.
- Able to think strategically.
- Are a risk taker (i.e. that you are able to move situations forward).

A dean would be expected to have substantial educational and research experience as well as a master's degree and a professional nursing qualification. Many deans now have doctorates and continue to be research active.

Educational support groups

There are several support groups available for those working in children's nursing education:

Royal College of Nursing (RCN)'s Children's Nursing Education Group (http://www2.rcn.org.uk/cyp/forums/rcn_professional_forums/childrens_nursing_education)

Association of British Paediatric Nurses Nurse Education Group (http://www.abpn.org.uk/site/nurse_education/294/nurse_education.aspx)

If you are a lecturer–practitioner, you might like to joint the National Lecturer Practitioner Forum (http://www.nlpf.org.uk/)

Career pathways in research

When considering a career in nursing research, it can be difficult to know where to start. The Scottish Executive and NHS Education for Scotland (2005) do provide some basic guidance for nurses, considering a career in research and emphasise the need to be proactive. Furthermore, the descriptions of the research careers of five nurses provided by Bishop (2004) suggest that many people find themselves in a research career almost by accident and as a result of a chance encounter or opportunity. Within this section, I will endeavour to provide some guidance for those wishing to pursue a career in nursing research.

Five potential career pathways: clinical research nurse, pharmaceutical, academic, management and clinical have been identified by the RCN's research society (Kenkre and Foxcroft 2001a, b, c, d, e).[1] Each career pathway has been presented as a matrix to demonstrate the facility to develop a career along a single pathway or by developing a greater knowledge by moving between pathways. The information provided includes the typical role, experience, knowledge, training, skills and qualifications expected at each stage along each pathway. The clinical research nurse, pharmaceutical and academic research pathways will be considered in detail. How the nurse working in clinical practice can be involved in research at the various stages of their career will also be discussed. Readers are referred to Kenkre and Foxcroft (2001d) for further information about the management pathway. [*Note*: Much of the information in this section is drawn from Kenkre and Foxcroft (2001a, b, c, e).]

Clinical research nurse career pathway

The role of the clinical research nurse is usually associated with working alongside medical staff in a clinical trial. Kenkre and Foxcroft (2001a) outline a career pathway for clinical research nurses. At each stage of the pathway, the clinical research nurse has more responsibility and increasing autonomy and research experience. To become a clinical research nurse, you need to have post-registration clinical experience within the speciality and be registered with the NMC. You may or may not have any research experience but should:

- Be numerate.
- Have good IT skills.
- Be able to adhere to a protocol.
- Be able to liaise with research staff and representatives of sponsor companies.
- Have good time management skills.
- Have project management skills.

A clinical research nurse in their first post will be expected to identify and screen suitable patients for trials and carry out procedures and treatment interventions according to pre-determined protocols. The clinical research nurse will be responsible for the day-to-day organisation of the trial, collection of data as well as data entry and patient support. For the clinical research nurse working with CYP, this may also reflect the need to support CYP in decisions around consent and involvement in research and also consideration of the needs of the family while following a research protocol.

To progress along the career pathway for clinical research nurses you will need to undertake additional training starting with a first degree and a certificate in clinical research and moving on to a masters degree in research methods and then an MBA or PhD. As your theoretical and practical knowledge increases, you will be able to move up the career pathway. The most senior clinical

---

[1]http://www.man.ac.uk/rcn/rs/career.htm (accessed 12 December 2006).

research nurse would be expected to have a doctorate and/or an MBA and be active at a national and international level.

The *International Conference on Harmonisation on Good Clinical Practice* (ICH GCP) sets out to provide a unified standard for the EU, Japan and the US to facilitate the mutual acceptance of clinical data by the regulatory authorities in these regions. Since 2005, EU Directive (2005/28/EC) has specified ICH GCP standards as a mandatory requirement for trials of investigational medical products. Undertaking a training course about these standards is essential for the clinical research nurse.

Pharmaceutical industry career pathway

Some nurses work in the pharmaceutical industry as clinical research associates, nurses who have previously worked in as specialist nurses with CYP such as with asthma, diabetes or epilepsy have found an interest in furthering their expertise through either research work or product development work. Nurses working in the pharmaceutical industry are usually involved in drug trials. According to Kenkre and Foxcroft (2001b), the trainee clinical research associate will:

- Perform monitoring visits with mentor to acquire the skills necessary to ensure that complete accurate data are retrieved from study sites.
- Complete independent ethics committee applications to gain insight into study protocol and design.
- Archive of trial master file data.

To become a *trainee clinical research associate*, you need a first degree (or higher) and/or a nursing background as well as some knowledge about the good clinical practice and the pharmaceutical industry. You will also need to be numerate, have good IT skills, be able to adhere to pre-determined protocols and able to liaise with research staff and other representatives. To advance along the career pathway to become a clinical research associate, you will need to consider undertaking a Certificate/Diploma in Clinical Research.

Once you have gained 6–12 months experience, you can apply for a *clinical research associate* post. You will then be expected to work on your own and be responsible for conducting monitoring visits and ensuring that data standards are met across all study sites. *Senior clinical research associates* have the additional responsibility of leading and managing teams. So to become a senior clinical research associate, you will need to undertake some management training. The final stage of the pharmaceutical industry pathway is to become a project manager or clinical research officer when you will be responsible for the strategic planning and financial management of the clinical trials process. At this level, you will be negotiated for contracts and need to be able to motivate and lead research teams and will usually have an MSc in clinical research. Undertaking ICH GCP training can also be seen to be essential for the nurse working in the pharmaceutical industry.

Academic research career pathway

The academic research career pathway is often seen as the traditional academic pathway. You can enter this pathway at a number of points. The first entry point is as a research assistant/research associate/research nurse. This position usually entails undertaking the practicalities a particular study, working to a research protocol organising and undertaking data collection, coding and entering data onto computer, and providing some input to preliminary data analysis and assisting with writing the reports and publications (Kenkre and Foxcroft 2001c). To become a research assistant/research associate/research nurse, having a first degree will be beneficial. You also need to:

- Be on the NMC register.
- Have post-registration clinical experience applicable to CYP nursing.
- Have an understanding of the importance of research within the health service.
- Have post-registration training in critical appraisal skills, audit and research methods.
- Have good IT skills.
- Be numerate.
- Be able to complete a literature review.
- Be able to work independently and as a team member.
- Have good time management skills.

Research assistant/research associate/research nurse appointments are often available as a secondment, at least in the short term, and so offer an opportunity to *test the waters* and see whether you are *cut out* to be a researcher.

The next step on the academic research career pathway is to become a *lecturer/research fellow*. Some people enter the academic research pathway at this point. These posts are usually a combined teaching and research role. The teaching may be related to clinical practice or research methods, whereas the research role involves working with more senior academics in the development of research protocols and in the preparation of reports and papers for publications (Kenkre and Foxcroft 2001c). For those working in the field of CYP research, specialist knowledge of the complexities of research with children and their families is important. Nurses working towards this role may come from various fields such as social work, health visiting, school nursing, child and adolescent mental health services (CAMHS) together with those from a traditional background of CYP nursing. To be offered a lecturer/research fellow post, you would be expected to have:

- Some experience of teaching and research.
- Some publications.
- Given several conferences papers.
- A master's degree with substantial research component such as a master's in research methods.

- Project management skills.
- Experience in protocol development and data analysis.

To be promoted to *senior (or principal) lecturer/senior research fellow*, you would be expected to have a doctorate and some post-doctoral experience. Senior (principal) lecturers/senior research fellows lead the development of projects and are active on research committees at a local and regional level. They will publish high-quality papers in a range of academic journals and apply for grants to bring in external research funding. Individuals in this role will often show initiative in terms of developing their own research agenda. At this level, you need to be able to lead and motivate a research team as well as have a comprehensive knowledge of the national R&D agenda.

Becoming a reader

Research active nurse academics who work primarily as lecturers or researchers can strive to become a *reader*. A reader is recognised as someone who has a robust research portfolio that demonstrates excellence and leadership in research. The criteria for appointment may vary slightly in each university but you would usually have a PhD and would also be expected to have:

- A track record of successful external grant application.
- A strong publication profile in academic journals.
- Presented a substantial number of conferences.
- Have a reputation as a leader in the field.
- Experience of supervising research projects.

Becoming a professor

Once you have become a reader you may want to aim to be promoted to become a *professor*. This is quite a recent progression for academics with the speciality of CYP nursing. If this is the case, you will need to have:

- A PhD in a relevant field and a post-doctoral track record.
- A proven track record in research.
- Been successful in securing research funding.
- Carried out pioneering research work.
- Experience of supervising research projects and students (preferably to include supervising PhD students to completion).
- Have international research collaborations.
- Excellent teaching skills.
- Proven qualities of academic leadership.
- The ability to think strategically.
- Experience of managing a team.

Support groups for nurse researchers

There are several support groups available for those working as nurse researcher or interested in developing their research skills:

- RCN's Research in Child Health (RiCH) Group (www.rcn.org.uk/rich)
- RCN's Research Society (http://www.man.ac.uk/rcn/rs/)

Clinical research nurses may wish to join the Clinical Research Nurses Association (www.man.ac.uk/rcn/ukwide/crna.htm).

Research and clinical practice

The different opportunities for clinical staff to be involved in research are outlined by Kenkre and Foxcroft (2001e). As a *staff nurse*, your role in research is likely to be limited, but there may be opportunities for you to become involved in research and audit. If you are interested in progressing along the career pathway to become a ward sister, clinical matron, nurse practitioner or nurse consultant, you should take advantage of any such opportunities that are on offer. You should also read and appraise the research-based literature relevant to your speciality. To be promoted within nursing, nowadays it is getting more and more important to have a degree. You should also join and participate in any relevant specialist interest groups within your place of work and at a national level (e.g. the RCN's forums and special interest groups). Joining such groups allows you to network with other people working in your speciality as well as ensuring that you stay up to date about current innovations.

Information about the RCN's forums and special interest groups can be found at: http://www2.rcn.org.uk/cyp/forums/rcn_professional_forums

---

The *ward manager, clinical matron* or *nurse practitioner* or *clinical nurse specialist's* role in research is primarily about ensuring that the research findings are integrated into patient care. Additionally, nurse practitioners or clinical nurse specialists may be involved in research studies either individually or as part of a team. Nurses working at this level will need to have a first degree and many nurses in these roles have master's degrees. Indeed, nurse practitioners and clinical nurse specialists will increasingly be expected to have a master's degree or even a doctorate.

The role of the nurse consultant in research and education

The role of the *nurse consultant* is discussed in Chapter 11. However, the a nurse consultant is expected to be competent in four core functions, one of which is practice and service development, research and evaluation, whereas another relates to education and training. To become a nurse consultant, you can expect, therefore, to have substantial experience in research, education and service development (Kenkre and Foxcroft 2001e).

The future for nursing academic careers

The publication of *Modernising Nursing Careers* (DH 2006) means that the future of nurse education and nursing itself will change over the next 5–10 years. Change is also afoot in relation to nursing clinical academic careers. As I write this chapter, the UK Clinical Research Collaboration (UKCRC) is deliberating about the future of nursing clinical academic career pathways. A look at their website indicates that they are working under the umbrella of the UKCRC Subcommittee; an Expert Reference Group has focused on a number of areas:

- Development of model pathways for early and mid career research nurses defined with multiple entry routes and levels of progress.
- Identification of support and training mechanisms.
- Testing of the models developed with a research nurse focus group.
- Examination of potential implementation processes and funding requirements.

(UKCRC 2006)

Further information can be found on the UKCRC website (www.ukcrc.org).

References

Bishop V (2004). Introduction to careers in nursing research: Case studies and opportunities. In: Freshwater D and Bishop V (eds), *Nursing Research in Context*, pp. 118–143. Basingstoke: Palgrave.

Department of Health (DH) (2006). *Modernising nursing careers: Setting the Direction*. London: The Stationery Office.

Directive 2005/28/EC of the European Parliament and the Council of 8 April 2005 laying down principles and detailed guidelines for good clinical practice as regards investigational medicinal products for human use, as well as the requirement for authorisation of the manufacturing or importation of such products.

Kenkre J and Foxcroft DR (2001a). Career pathways in research: Clinical research. *Nursing Standard*, 16(5), 41–44.

Kenkre J and Foxcroft DR (2001b). Career pathways in research: Pharmaceutical. *Nursing Standard*, 16(8), 36–39.

Kenkre J and Foxcroft DR (2001c). Career pathways in research: Academic. *Nursing Standard*, 16(7), 40–44.

Kenkre J and Foxcroft DR (2001d). Career pathways in research: Support and management. *Nursing Standard*, 16(6), 33–35.

Kenkre J and Foxcroft DR (2001e). Career pathways in research: Clinical practice. *Nursing Standard*, 16(4), 40–43.

Kingston University (2001). *Academic Salary Progression and Promotion*. London: Kingston University.

Leigh J, Howarth M and Devitt P (2005). The role of the lecturer practitioner: An exploration of the stakeholders and practitioners perspective. *Nurse Education in Practice*, 5, 258–265.

Rhead M and Strange F (1996). Nursing lecturer/practitioners: Can lecturer/practitioners be music to our ears. *Journal of Advanced Nursing*, 24, 1265–1272.

Scottish Executive and NHS Education for Scotland (2005). *Making Choices, Facing Challenges: Developing Your Research Career in Nursing, Midwifery and the Allied Health Professions*. Edinburgh: Scottish Executive.

UKCRC (2006). http://www.ukcrc.org/activities/researchworkforce.aspx (accessed 15 December 2006).

University of Hertfordshire (2006). *Research and Scholarly Activity (Self Managed)*. http://perseus.herts.ac.uk/administration/personnel/website/a-zinfo/hourswrkdirectivs/reschschactivity.cfm (accessed 13 November 2006).

Chapter 13
Looking to the Future

Peter Callery

I have a copy of a textbook on diseases of infancy and childhood from the middle of the past century that makes interesting and sometimes comic reading (Sheldon 1946). There are substantial sections devoted to infectious diseases that are either no longer seen at all or only very rarely in western countries, including smallpox, poliomyelitis and diphtheria, reminding us of the enormous benefits brought by immunisation in the intervening years. Similarly, some modern terminology does not appear in Sheldon's book, for example there is no reference to bronchiolitis in the index. Changes in the understanding of diseases are illustrated by the limited attention given to mental health problems, which include 'hysteria' – a diagnosis that would not be recognised today. No doubt in 60 years, the cutting-edge textbooks of today will seem just as quaint and antiquated.

Looking ahead is fraught with difficulty because what seems important now may become irrelevant as new technologies or social changes shape the future. However, there are trends in childhood illness, in the organisation of services and the development of new nursing roles that can be expected to continue in the coming years. There are opportunities for imaginative and creative nurses to contribute even more to improve children's health in the future.

Changing perspectives on childhood

Recent decades have seen a major change in attitudes towards children and their development. For a long time, the seminal work of Piaget had dominated our understanding of child development and in particular cognitive development. This approach to child development has more recently been criticised for concentrating on deficits rather than abilities. There has also been increased interest in agency in childhood, which means considering children as people in their own right who act to create their own worlds and relationships rather than as passive 'proto-adults' who only become real people once they have grown to adulthood. A new sociology of childhood has grown up around these ideas (James 1993, James and Prout 1997). Concepts of children as people with rights are also reflected in policy debates at both the international level with the promulgation of the United Nations convention on the rights of the child (UNICEF

1990) and the national level with children's involvement in choices and decisions about their own care highlighted in the National Service Framework (Department of Health and Department for Education and Skills 2004).

Child and family-centred care

The term 'family-centred care' is frequently used in children's nursing to encompass concepts of parental participation in children's health care; partnership and collaboration between the health care team and parents in decision making; family friendly environments that normalise as much as possible family functioning within the health care setting and care of family members as well as of children (Franck and Callery 2004). The value of the concepts of family-centred care continues to be identified. One example – since parents' mental health problems can also impact on child development, there is a strong case for considering 'a child's development in the context of the whole family, rather than in isolation' (Blair and Hall 2006). However, the extent to which the concepts are supported by research and applied in practice remains unclear. The challenge remains to produce creative changes to the organisation and delivery of services, so that the concepts of child and family-centred care are operationalised in practice. Research is needed to understand the perspectives of children and their families, to identify how best to involve children and families in planning and providing care and how to assess family-centred care in practice.

Individualisation, choice, involvement and information

Information and involvement in decisions was identified as an area that demonstrated considerable room for improvement in the 2004 Patient Survey of 62,277 young people (response rate 50%) treated as inpatients in 150 National Health Service (NHS) acute and specialist trusts. The survey found that 'just under a third of parents said they were not involved as much as they wanted to be in decisions about the young patients' care and treatment. Forty-seven per cent of young patients said they were not involved in decisions as much as they wanted to be during their hospital stay' (Healthcare Commission 2005). Young patients were less likely than parents to report that they received information about their care and treatment in a way they could understand: 57% of young patients reported that doctors definitely gave them such information and a further 33% had this information from doctors to some extent (Healthcare Commission 2005, p. 13). Self-care information is particularly important given the short length of most childhood hospitalisations, but the survey suggested that parents and children did not receive complete information. Although almost all sent home with medication were given enough information about how to use it, only 51% of patients were given a full explanation of possible side effects, with 18% having some explanation and 31% no explanation about side effects (Healthcare Commission 2005, p. 16). 'Most young patients were given some information about danger signals to watch for when at home and when they could carry on with normal activities such as playing sport. However, 14% did not receive any information about danger signals and 16% did not receive information about resuming normal activities' (Healthcare Commission 2005, p. 16). Since the survey only sampled children and young people admitted to hospital, it does not provide information about the experiences of young people cared for in the community. However, there is evidence that children do not have the information they need to live with chronic illness. Children and young people with asthma were invited to complete a survey through the Blue Peter website in 2005 (Asthma UK 2006). More than half of the 17,340 respondents said that asthma placed limitations on their lives. Asthma had given 58% problems sleeping or prevented them from doing everyday activities within the last month. Although 55% of the children felt that their asthma was under control, more than one-third of these children were using their reliever inhalers >3 times a week, suggesting inadequate control (British Thoracic Society and Scottish Intercollegiate Guidelines Network 2003). Part of the explanation for this poor level of control was that 36% said that they did not know or were unsure how their preventer inhaler helps their asthma. Only 15% reported that they had a written personal asthma action plan as recommended for everyone with asthma (British Thoracic Society and Scottish Intercollegiate Guidelines Network 2003). Worryingly, 32% said that they did not know what to do if they had an asthma attack.

The need for clear communication of information to children and their families will grow as treatments advance and more choices are available. The surveys above suggest that there is already a major need for improvement in the way that information is provided and children and their families are involved in decisions about care. These issues will be an important part of the future of children's health care. Nurses should be well positioned to respond to the concerns of children and parents. It is very often nurses who are the principal information providers, interpreting and clarifying the information given to children and their families by other health professionals, and responding to questions as they arise. The evidence of the surveys by the Healthcare Commission and Asthma UK, should therefore be of particular concern to nursing. Research is needed to tell us whether nurses need more skills, more time or changed attitudes if communication is to be improved. There is evidence that children can identify the information that they want to receive about their health care and that they are interested enough to seek out information in whatever form available – even if this means using information provided for adults that may not be particularly well designed or appropriate for children (Smith and Callery 2005).

The potential to provide children, young people and their families with information through the Internet is far from realised. The Children First website gives children direct access to age-specific information (http://www.childrenfirst.nhs.uk/), and there are lively sites designed for teenagers such as Teenage Health Freak (http://www.teenagehealthfreak.org). As technology develops, there will be new opportunities to personalise information to the needs of individual children and their families. Nurses with the right technical and creative support could make exciting websites that would really help children and young people to understand their conditions and make the best choices about health care. Research is needed to identify the information needs of children with specific conditions, which might differ from the information needs of parents and other family members, and to identify the most appropriate formats and uses of technology to communicate health information.

Early intervention to address early disadvantage

Early disadvantage can have major health implications throughout life, suggesting the importance of early intervention to improve the prospects of children who start life in deprived circumstances. There is evidence from the US that programmes such as Head Start can be effective in 'preventing developmental delay, as assessed by reductions in retention in grade and placement in special education' (Anderson *et al*. 2003). Given the complexity of the problems associated with early disadvantage including children's own characteristics as well as those of their families and the social environment in which they live (Anderson *et al*. 2003), it is unrealistic to expect that brief interventions focused on single problems can do much to protect children against the cumulative factors that can negatively influence development (Blair and Hall 2006). Integration of health, education, and social services expertise is needed to address obstacles to optimum child development including 'the social and mental health issues affecting parents and carers, the difficulties that many adults have in understanding the needs of young children, and the poverty of learning opportunities experienced by many children' (Blair and Hall 2006). Nurses and health visitors have important contributions to make if they can work effectively within multi-disciplinary and multi-agency teams. Co-ordination of the efforts of education, health and social care agencies is therefore key to the development of effective interventions to improve children's life chances.

Particular skill and attention is required to make interventions accessible to the children who need them most because 'those families who might benefit the most are the ones least likely to access such help' (Blair and Hall 2006). The national evaluation of Sure Start Local Programmes (SSLP) has found that 'parents/families with greater human capital were better able to take advantage of SSLP services and resources than those with less human capital (i.e. teen parents, lone parents, workless households)', and previous studies have also found that interventions can produce greater benefits for the moderately than for the more severely disadvantaged (National Evaluation of Sure Start Team 2005). This suggests that special skills are required to assist the most disadvantaged families to make best use of the services that are available to them. Nurses and health visitors who are skilled in communicating and engaging with such families could make a significant contribution to child health by designing and marketing services that the hardest to reach groups in society will use. Research is needed to identify the hidden barriers that limit access of such families to effective services and into how best health professionals can help maximise the benefits for children and families.

Early detection of disabling conditions

Pre-school children are at risk of difficulties in speech and language development, general and specific learning disabilities, co-ordination problems, emotional and behavioural disorders. It has been suggested that the overall prevalence of such problems is between 10 and 20% (Blair and Hall 2006), which if correct suggests that they constitute a major health problem. These are difficult conditions to detect and diagnose because often 'they lie on a continuum of ability rather than reflecting a specific deficit or defect, so it is difficult to define what does or does not constitute a problem' (Blair and Hall 2006). As our expectations of health increase with overall improvements in child health, there will be less tolerance of problems that may have received less attention in the past. The grey area at the margin between clearly defined disability and what is considered within normal limits will become more difficult to identify. Such problems are usually first noticed by parents although there can be long delays before appropriate referral and intervention (Rannard *et al.* 2005). Nurses and health visitors are well placed to contribute to early detection. Parents may raise their concerns if given opportunities to talk about their children's development during encounters with health visitors and nurses. To identify cases of genuine concern and to distinguish from the 'worried well', nurses and health visitors will need the skills to interpret parents' lay knowledge, which is based on the experience of living with a child and to bridge the gap with professional knowledge which emphasises objective assessment against diagnostic criteria. Research is needed to help primary care practitioners identify the signs that parents notice and how these can guide professionals to make early, appropriate referrals of children who require assistance.

Mental health

Mental health problems are common in childhood: 'One in ten children in Great Britain aged 5–16 had a clinically recognisable mental disorder in 2004' (Office for National Statistics 2005). Social changes are associated with increased mental health problems. Changes in the structure of families and unemployment are two factors associated with increased difficulty for children. Mental health problems are more common among children in lone parent families (16%) than those in two-parent families (8%) and in families with neither parent working (20%) compared with those in which both parents work (8%). It appears then that mental health problems of children are associated with stresses in the lives of their families. Although the UK annual divorce rate dropped by 8% in 2005 to 13 per 1000 of the married population (Office for National Statistics 2006), it can be expected that a large proportion of children will be living with only one parent in the future, thus placing them at greater risk of mental health problems. Unemployment is at a historically low level, although with a rising trend at the time of writing, and there are ~2 million people in the UK not working due to long-term illness. Future increases in unemployment and/or disability could further add to the burden of mental health problems in childhood.

The number of children and young people seen by Child and Adolescent Mental Health Services (CAMHS) has been rising in recent years although the number of new cases means that there have also been increases in those waiting up to 6 months (Barnes *et al.* 2006), which is a long time for a child or young person with a mental health problem that could be affecting emotional, social, physical, cognitive and educational development.

Nurses outside as well as inside CAMHS could contribute to early detection and intervention of mental health problems. There is great potential to develop school-based initiatives that promote self-help among children and young people to prevent problems becoming more serious and affecting healthy development. Research is needed to examine what support could be most useful to children and young people and how services could be integrated into schools as well as primary care.

Hospital and home care

Part of the vision of the National Service Framework for Children and Young People (NSF Standard 6) is to see: 'Children and young people who are ill receiving timely, high quality and effective care as close to home as possible' (Department of Health and Department for Education and Skills 2004). Services should therefore be designed to limit hospital attendance to those occasions when care cannot be provided in the community. However, non-surgical paediatric admissions and Accident and Emergency department (A&E) attendances are still rising albeit at a slower pace than in the early 1990s (Armon *et al.* 2001, MacFaul and Werneke 2001), and there has been 'a substantial shift of work from general practice to hospital, although this is difficult to quantify' (Craft 2004). Emergency care in hospitals could be used by parents because out of hours services such as NHS Direct often direct parents to a primary care assessment facility or a hospital emergency department (Hall and Sowden 2005). Presentation by children to emergency services for minor illnesses can lead to inappropriate admission to hospital (MacFaul *et al.* 1994, Stewart *et al.* 1998). Observation and Assessment Units (OAUs) have been developed to provide a setting where children can be observed and assessed by experienced medical and nursing staff for a limited number of hours and safely sent home, thus avoiding unnecessary admission (Lamireau *et al.* 2000, Aitken *et al.* 2003, Zebrack *et al.* 2005). Different models of OAUs have developed, variously described as emergency assessment, observation, or short stay units. Some are situated in A&E departments, whereas others are based on near Children's Wards. Ambulatory services also include acute assessment clinics based in outpatient departments. A systematic review identified 13 studies of acute assessment units based in paediatric departments, 9 study units based in A&E departments and 3 studies of acute assessment clinics (Ogilvie 2005). About 40% of children attending acute assessment units in paediatric departments and over 60% of those attending acute assessment units in A&E departments were discharged, suggesting that they did not require inpatient admission. Although there were methodological problems with many studies, the limited evidence available suggests that OAUs can be safe, efficient, and acceptable alternatives to inpatient admission (Ogilvie 2005). OAUs are likely to become an increasingly important part of children's health care, because they give parents quick access to confident, credible paediatric advice. OAUs will be attractive to health service managers if they are demonstrated to reduce the need for short-term admissions. Nurse practitioners and nurse consultants have been proposed as the key frontline staff for OAUs by leading paediatricians (Craft 2004). There is a great opportunity for children's nurses to assess children in OAUs, identifying when admission is required and giving parents the information to enable them to care for their children safely at home.

OAUs may be at their most effective when operating in conjunction with home nursing by Community Children's Teams (CCTs). Recent years have seen a substantial increase in paediatric home care services. The Royal College of Nursing (RCN) listed 27 services in its first directory of community children's nursing teams in 1987, whereas ~240 services were included in the 2005 version (Whiting 2006). However, development of services has occurred on an *ad hoc* basis, which has led to considerable diversity in CCT provision (Eaton 2000). Most are based in hospitals although approximately a quarter are managed and/or based in community settings. They vary widely in size, from single nurses to teams numbering at least 20 nurses (While and Dyson 2000). A national survey in 2001 reported that children's hospital at home or home nursing services differed by trust affiliation, staffing, skill mix, caseload, procedures undertaken and hours of operation. Some teams had a predominantly acute caseload, whereas others dealt with a mixture of acute and chronic cases or with predominantly chronic cases (Cramp *et al.* 2003).

Differences in the organisation of CCTs have implications for the delivery of care to children. Community-based and community-managed CCTs may be better placed to develop links with primary health care and other local health and social care services (While and Dyson 2000). Hospital-based and hospital-managed CCTs may have stronger links to acute services, for example in some services staff rotate between home and ward nursing. However, comparative evidence is lacking because evaluation of CCTs has been conducted at the local level. Typically, studies have compared satisfaction with, and safety of, single home nursing services with hospital care for children with acute illnesses. A randomised controlled trial of a paediatric hospital at home scheme suggested that children with acute medical conditions can be safely managed at home and that home care is preferred by parents and children because it is less socially disruptive and avoids the financial costs associated with hospitalisation (Sartain *et al.* 2002). Another evaluation found that a service for children with acute conditions led to a reduction in admissions and length of stay and that professionals and parents were positive to the introduction of the service (Davies and Dale 2003a, b). A systematic review for the Health Technology Assessment programme reported that all the studies of paediatric acute home care are small-scale studies of single teams operating within a particular local context, which makes systematic comparison and generalisability problematic (Parker *et al.* 2002). The review also noted that the research evidence on the cost-effectiveness of paediatric home care is weak with few studies directly comparing the delivery of hospital services with home care or comparing different models of home care. Because service models have developed at the local level, a complex pattern of different models of CCT and OAUs has emerged. Research is required to assess the relative effectiveness of different models of both CCTs and OAUs. It would be particularly valuable for research to examine the interaction between CCTs and OAUs – for example to test whether discharge from OAUs to home care supported by a CCT can reduce the number of inappropriate admissions while providing parents and children with safe and care that meets their needs.

Health technology

As health care improves, a growing number of children are living at home with a continuing need for the support of medical technology. Families living in this situation face many difficulties, including obtaining appropriate and co-ordinated home support services. The key worker concept is particularly important for such families, and it can be expected that there will be increasing demands on nurses to develop the skills and networks to work in co-ordination with colleagues from other helping professions across social and educational as well as health care agencies. Living with technology dependence also places strain on family relationships. Parents can feel conflicts between their roles as nurturing, supportive parents and the demands of medical technology, which can make them feel like 'nurses' to their children (Kirk *et al.* 2005). More families will be facing such issues as new technologies are introduced into the care of children in their homes, and they will look for nurses to help them to cope with the psychosocial consequences of caring for technology-dependent children as well as training in the use of equipment.

Advanced practice

There are many opportunities for nurses to develop new roles in children's health care in the future. The concept of advanced practice roles has been proven in posts developed to substitute for doctors in hospital settings where medical staffing has been reduced as a result of legislation on working hours. Paediatric nurse practitioners were among the first nurses to take on advanced roles in the US. The economics of medical staffing have often determined the extension of nursing roles. The US experience suggests that there is potential for children's nurses to develop advanced practice in community settings in the UK as part of a reconfiguration of general practice. Such roles would require nurse practitioners to have good knowledge of local determinants of health within communities, making it possible to support the child and family beyond the treatment of presenting complaints (Hall and Lawson 2004). Nurses could learn much from health visitors who have developed skills in working with communities as well as individuals, using public health concepts and methods.

Education

It has been suggested that general practitioner education will have to respond to the expectations of children and parents: 'Tomorrow's parents and young people will expect their doctor to have confirmed competences in acute and non-urgent children's care, particularly psychological disorders and chronic disease' (Hall and Sowden 2005). Nurses are likely to meet similar expectations. As children and parents increasingly need interventions that help them to address their psychological concerns and to care for chronic conditions, nurses will require the skills and knowledge to further develop their educational roles with children and families.

References

Aitken P, Birch S, Cogman G, Glasper EA and Wiltshire M (2003). Quadrennial review of a paediatric emergency assessment unit. *British Journal of Nursing*, 12(4), 234–241.

Anderson LM, Shinn C, Fullilove MT, Scrimshaw SC, Fielding JE, Normand J, Carande-Kulis VG and Task Force on Community Preventive Services (2003). The effectiveness of early childhood development programs. A systematic review [see comment]. *American Journal of Preventive Medicine*, 24(3 Suppl), 32–46.

Armon K, Stephenson T, Gabriel V, MacFaul R, Eccleston P, Werneke U and Smith S (2001). Determining the common medical presenting problems to an accident and emergency department. *Archives of Disease in Childhood*, 84(5), 390–392.

Asthma UK (2006). Blue Peter survey results. Asthma UK, Web page.

Barnes D, Wistow R, Dean R and Foster B (2006). National Child and Adolescent Mental Health Service Mapping Exercise 2005.

Blair M and Hall D (2006). From health surveillance to health promotion: The changing focus in preventive children's services. *Archives of Disease in Childhood*, 91(9), 730–735.

British Thoracic Society and Scottish Intercollegiate Guidelines Network (2003). British guideline on the management of asthma. *Thorax*, 58(Suppl 1), i1–i94.

Craft A (2004). Out of hours care. *Archives of Disease in Childhood*, 89(2), 112–113.

Cramp C, Tripp S and Dale J (2003). Children's home nursing: Results of a national survey. *Paediatric Nursing*, 15(8), 39–43.

Davies C and Dale J (2003a). Paediatric home care for acute illness: I. GPs' and hospital-at-home staff views. *International Journal of Health Care Quality Assurance*, 16(6/7), 361–366.

Davies C and Dale J (2003b). Paediatric home care for acute illness: III. Parental views. *International Journal of Health Care Quality Assurance*, 16(5), 229–233.

Department of Health and Department for Education and Skills (2004). *National Service Framework for Children, Young People and Maternity Services*. London.

Eaton N (2000). Children's community nursing services: Models of care delivery. A review of the United Kingdom literature. *Journal of Advanced Nursing*, 32(1), 49–56.

Franck LS and Callery P (2004). Re-thinking family-centred care across the continuum of children's healthcare. *Child: Care, Health and Development*, 30(3), 265–277.

Hall D and Sowden D (2005). Primary care for children in the 21st century. *British Medical Journal*, 330(7489), 430–431.

Hall S and Lawson C (2004). Nurse practitioners [see comment]. *Archives of Disease in Childhood*, 89(2), 118–119.

Healthcare Commission (2005). *Patient Survey Report 2004 – Young Patients*. Healthcare Commission, London.

James A (1993). *Childhood Identities: Self and Social Relationships in the Experience of the Child*. Edinburgh: Edinburgh University Press.

James A and Prout A (eds) (1997). *Constructing and Reconstructing Childhood: Contemporary Issues in the Sociological Study of Childhood*. London: Falmer Press.

Kirk S, Glendinning C and Callery P (2005). Parent or nurse? The experience of being the parent of a technology-dependent child. *Journal of Advanced Nursing*, 51(5), 456–464.

Lamireau T, Llanas B, Dommange S, Genet C and Fayon M (2000). A short-stay observation unit improves care in the paediatric emergency care setting [see comment]. *European Journal of Emergency Medicine*, 7(4), 261–265.

MacFaul R and Werneke U (2001). Recent trends in hospital use by children in England. *Archives of Disease in Childhood*, 85(3), 203–207.

MacFaul R, Glass EJ and Jones S (1994). Appropriateness of paediatric admission. *Archives of Disease in Childhood*, 71(1), 50–58.

National Evaluation of Sure Start Team (2005). *Early Impacts of Sure Start Local Programmes on Children and Families – Full Report*. Institute for the Study of Children, Families & Social Issues, Birkbeck, University of London, London.

Office for National Statistics (2005). *Mental Health: 1 in 10 Children has a Mental Disorder*. ONS. National Statistics London.

Office for National Statistics (2006). Divorce. Office for National Statistics; General Register Office for Scotland, Northern Ireland Statistics and Research Agency. http://www.statistics.gov.uk/cci/nugget.asp?id=170

Ogilvie D (2005). Hospital based alternatives to acute paediatric admission: A systematic review. *Archives of Disease in Childhood*, 90(2), 138–142.

Parker G, Bhakta P, Lovett C, Paisley S, Olsen R, Turner D and Young B (2002). A systematic review of the costs and effectiveness of different models of paediatric home care. *Health Technology Assessment*, 6(35).

Rannard A, Lyons C and Glenn S (2005). Parent concerns and professional responses: The case of specific language impairment. *British Journal of General Practice*, 55(518), 710–714.

Sartain SA, Maxwell MJ, Todd PJ, Jones KH, Bagust A, Haycox A and Bundred P (2002). Randomised controlled trial comparing an acute paediatric hospital at home scheme with conventional hospital care. *Archives of Disease in Childhood*, 87(5), 371–375.

Sheldon W (1946). *Diseases of Infancy and Childhood*. London: J. & A. Churchill Ltd.

Smith L and Callery P (2005). Children's accounts of their preoperative information needs. *Journal of Clinical Nursing*, 14(2), 230–238.

Stewart U, Werneke R, MacFaul R, Taylor Meek J, Smith HE and Smith IJ (1998). Medical and social factors associated with the admission and discharge of acutely ill children. *Archives of Disease in Childhood*, 79(3), 219–224.

UNICEF (1990). *Office of the United Nations High Commissioner for Human Rights (OHCHR)*. Geneva, Switzerland: UNICEF.

While AE and Dyson L (2000). Characteristics of paediatric home care provision: The two dominant models in England. *Child: Care, Health and Development*, 26(4), 263–276.

Whiting M (2006). *Directory of Community Children's Nursing Services*, Vol. 2005. Royal College of Nursing Community Children's Nursing Forum, http://wwwirch.org.uk/development/communities/specialisms/community/childrens_nursing/directory

Zebrack M, Kadish H and Nelson D (2005). The pediatric hybrid observation unit: An analysis of 6477 consecutive patient encounters. *Pediatrics*, 115(5), e535–e542.

Index